Case Presentations in Clinical Infections

Ian K. Hosein   MB BCH Dip Am Board Path FCAP MRCPath
Consultant Medical Microbiologist
Department of Medical Microbiology and Public Health Laboratory
University Hospital of Wales
Cardiff
UK

Meirion B. Llewelyn   BSc MB BCH Phd MRCP
Senior Registrar in Respiratory Medicine
Department of Medicine
University Hospital of Wales
Cardiff
UK

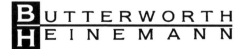

BUTTERWORTH
HEINEMANN

Butterworth-Heinemann
Linacre House, Jordan Hill, Oxford OX2 8DP
A division of Reed Educational and Professional Publishing Ltd

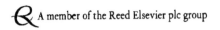 A member of the Reed Elsevier plc group

OXFORD   BOSTON   JOHANNESBURG

MELBOURNE   NEW DELHI   SINGAPORE

First published 1997

British Library Cataloguing in Publication Data
A catalogue record for this book is available from the British Library

Library of Congress Cataloguing in Publication Data
A catalogue record for this book is available from the Library of Congress

ISBN 0 7506 2184 2

Typeset by Bath Typesetting
Printed and bound in Great Britain by Biddles Ltd, Guildford and King's Lynn

Case Presentations in Clinical Infections

Titles in the series

Contents

Preface

This collection of cases gives a practical approach to infection covering a breadth of organisms, organ systems and syndromes. Whilst principally directed at those studying for higher qualifications in medicine, infectious diseases, public health medicine and medical microbiology, the book will also be of help to undergraduates, since core principles are equally applicable. The cases can 'stand alone'; however, optimal gain will be achieved if in-depth study is pursued by referring to relevant textbooks and original articles.

We wish to thank Neil Carbans for his help in proof-reading many of the Case Studies.

Ian K. Hosein and Meirion B. Llewelyn

Case 1   Legal action for hospital-acquired infection

A 25-year-old woman presented at term for elective lower segment Caesarean section because of breech presentation. This was her first pregnancy and she had been very well with an uneventful past history. The operation lasted 30 min and was performed under routine surgical conditions with one obstetric registrar, one senior house officer, one scrubbed midwife and one anaesthetic senior house officer in attendance. Two doses of cefuroxime 750 mg i.v. were given as antibiotic prophylaxis, starting immediately pre-operatively. On the second post-operative day she became febrile and had a purulent vaginal discharge. Cefuroxime and metronidazole were given i.v. but there was continued deterioration over the next 48 h. A swab of the discharge grew *Staphylococcus aureus* and antimicrobial sensitivities were pending. A microbiology registrar fortuitously suggested adding systemic vancomycin and she made a rapid recovery. The *S. aureus* isolated was unexpectedly methicillin resistant. The patient is deeply concerned that she may have acquired this organism in hospital.

Questions

1. What defence can a hospital mount in the face of litigation for presumed hospital acquired infection from, say, methicillin-resistant *Staphylococcus aureus* (MRSA)?
2. If you advocate prophylaxis covering *S. aureus* in this or any other operation, when would you consider cover for MRSA?
3. What is the significance of hyperbetalactamase producing *S. aureus*?

Answers

1. Litigation for presumed hospital-acquired infection is increasing and, with the now widespread occurrence of MRSA, frequently involves this organism. A well organized Infection Prevention and Control Programme will reduce the spread of this and other pathogens and demonstrates organizational

commitment. Such a programme should include evidence of staff education for implementation of infection prevention and control policies and effective surveillance systems for sporadic infection and outbreaks.

2. This question may be asked with regard to any organism with a resistant population and also has implications for empirical therapy of infections. With the inactivity of beta-lactam agents against MRSA, the use of common prophylactics such as cefuroxime or flucloxacillin would be very risky indeed in a patient at risk of MRSA infection. If the patient is a known MRSA carrier or if the overall rate of MRSA amongst all *S. aureus* isolates is rising, say, to 10%, one should consider prophylaxis with vancomycin or teicoplanin where staphylococcal prophylaxis is needed.

3. Hyperbetalactamase producing *S. aureus* may appear to be resistant to methicillin because of very large-scale production of β-lactamase but they are not resistant *in vivo*. Reduction of MICs or increase in zone sizes by the addition of a betalactamase inhibitor such as clavulanate can be used *in vitro* to demonstrate sensitivity to methicillin. Infections with these strains can therefore be treated with amoxycillin-clavulanate (co-amoxiclav), flucloxacillin or cefuroxime.

Comment

An exact figure of when to consider increased cover because of a resistant population cannot be given. The 10% mentioned in this case is meant to provoke thought on the issues involved, such as wound infection rate and consequences of such infection.

Hyperbetalactamase-producing strains are mentioned again to provoke thought because of the plethora of adjectives now relating to the resistance of *S. aureus* such as 'penicillinase producing', 'methicillin-resistant', 'epidemic methicillin-resistant', 'oxacillin-resistant' etc. The present confusion over MRSA observed on wards in part arises from these multiple terms and particularly when strain behaviour is related to resistance. For example, certain strains of MRSA (as indeed any *S. aureus*) may behave more aggressively (faster spread or more invasive disease) regardless of specific resistance to, say, gentamicin or fucidin, but how a given strain will behave when first detected on a ward cannot be reliably predicted. Standard control measures must therefore be employed for all MRSA; other measures may be stepped up or down depending on subsequently observed behaviour.

Further reading

WORKING PARTY OF THE HOSPITAL INFECTION SOCIETY AND BRITISH SOCIETY FOR ANTIMICROBIAL CHEMOTHERAPY (1990) Revised guidelines for the control of epidemic methicillin-resistant *Staphylococcus aureus*. *J. Hosp. Infect.*, **16**, 351–377.
ZIERDT, C., HOSEIN, I., SHIVELY, R. AND MacLOWRY, J. (1992) Phage pattern specific oxacillin-resistant and borderline oxacillin-resistant *Staphylococcus aureus* in U.S. hospitals – epidemiological significance. *J. Clin. Microbiol.*, **30**, 252–254.
KEANE, C. T., COLEMAN, D. C. AND CAFFERKEY, M. T. (1991) Methicillin-resistant *Staphylococcus aureus* – a reappraisal. *J. Hosp. Infect.*, **19**, 147–152.

Case 2   Cystic structures in broncho-alveolar lavage fluid

A 38-year-old town planner was admitted to hospital with left-sided chest pains. He had been well up until 3 weeks earlier when he suffered rigors followed by persistent malaise. Four days before admission he developed shortness of breath, cough productive of green sputum, left-side pleuritic chest pains and also complained of a slight headache. He was seen by his general practitioner who prescribed erythromycin but the symptoms did not resolve and he was referred to hospital.

He had stopped smoking 15 cigarettes a day 2 months previously, and had no history of pulmonary disease. He was homosexual, living with the same partner for 5 years. The partner was known to be negative for human immunodeficiency virus (HIV).

On admission the patient was breathless and febrile (38°C) and was noted to have seborrhoeic dermatitis over the forehead and eyebrows. There was oral candidiasis. The neck was not stiff; and several pea-sized lymph nodes were palpated in the cervical region. Fundoscopy was normal. Examination of the chest revealed basal crackles on the left-side only. The haemoglobin was 11.4 g/dl and the white blood count was 19.3×10^9/l. The blood gases were PO_2 63 mmHg, PCO_2 30 mmHg, pH 7.41., and a chest

X-ray showed an area of confluent consolidation in the left mid-zone. His mucopurulent sputum yielded no significant pathogens on routine Gram staining and culture but bronchoalveolar lavage showed numerous cystic structures, 6 microns in diameter after staining with Grocott's methenamine silver.

Questions

1. What other investigations should be performed on the lavage specimen?
2. What other laboratory tests are indicated?

Answers

1. Further investigations on the lavage specimen should be:
   (i) Immunofluorescent antibody staining for *Pneumocystis carinii;*
   (ii) Staining and culture for acid-fast bacilli;
   (iii) Gram stain and bacterial cultures (including for Legionella);
   (iv) Wet preparation and inoculation of fungal culture media for fungi;
   (v) Direct fluorescent antibody staining for respiratory viruses and viral culture;
2. Useful blood tests would include:
   (i) Human immunodeficiency virus serology (following informed consent);
   (ii) Legionella antibody and cryptococcal antigen titre in serum should be considered.

Comment

This patient is homosexual with a pneumonia and the acquired immune deficiency syndrome (AIDS) should be considered at presentation. Other features suggestive of HIV infection in this case were oral candidiasis and seborrhoeic dermatitis. Lymphadenopathy is a variable finding and the disappearance of previously large lymph nodes is a bad prognostic sign.

The approach to the patient with pulmonary disease who is at risk of HIV infection is guided by the types and frequency of pulmonary disorders reported in the literature on such patients; 85% will have *Pneumocystis* pneumonia with or without other pathogens. Other primary pathogens are *Mycobacterium aviumintracellulare*, pyogenic bacteria (especially *S. pneumoniae* and *H. influenzae*), legionella, cryptococcus, *M. tuberculosis*, Herpes simplex and *Toxoplasma gondii*. Non-infectious disorders can also occur; Kaposi's sarcoma in 5%, and non-Hodgkin's lymphoma in 2%. Cytomegalovirus (CMV) pneumonia is a controversial issue. Only by biopsy material can the involvement of CMV be ascertained, as shedding of CMV in sputum and urine is virtually universal in persons infected with HIV.

The first fact to establish is whether or not *Pneumocystis carinii* is present. In some units sputum induced following administration of nebulized 3% saline is examined. This saves the patient being lavaged if positive, but a negative result cannot be regarded as definitive. Units with bronchoscopic facilities often perform bronchoalveolar lavage (BAL) which has been reported to have a sensitivity for *P. carinii* of 97%. *P. carinii* cannot be grown in the clinical laboratory and direct examination of a lavage concentrate with immunofluorescent monoclonal antibody staining is used. Such staining distinguishes *P. carinii* from fungi such as *Cryptococcus neoformans* which also stains with Grocott's methenamine silver. In this case such antibody staining was negative and subsequently *Cryptococcus neoformans* was grown from BAL fluid, blood and cerebrospinal fluid.

Cryptococcus neoformans is an encapsulated yeast most commonly found in soil contaminated with bird droppings and is contracted by inhalation. Cryptococcus is the fourth most common cause of serious disease in AIDS patients after *P. carinii*, CMV and mycobacteria. Although cryptococcus was grown from CSF, the patient did not have meningism or photophobia in common with 70% of AIDS patients with cryptococcal meningitis.

Treatment choice depends on whether the patient is in a high or low risk prognostic category judged by CSF cryptococcal antigen titre, level of consciousness and CSF white cell count. Patients in the high risk group are treated with amphotericin B with or without flucytosine and those in the low risk group with fluconazole. Oral fluconazole is continued indefinitely after the acute illness to suppress cryptococcus, which cannot be completely eradicated from tissue such as the prostate.

Further reading

LEVITZ, S. M. (1991) The ecology of *Cryptococcus neoformans* and the epidemiology of cryptococcosis. *Rev. Infect. Dis.*, **13**, 1163–1169.

Case 3   Bacteraemia following a seafood meal

A 55-year-old female with a long-standing history of alcoholic liver disease travelled from the United Kingdom to Florida for a holiday. Whilst there, she had a seafood meal which included raw oysters. Over the next 24 h she developed a fever, vomiting and increasing abdominal pain. She was rushed to the nearest hospital by her husband and collapsed in transit. On admission the patient was shocked with a blood pressure of 90/60 mmHg; temperature 38.4°C, respiratory rate 25/min and heart rate 96/min. Because of the history (as obtained from her husband) and clinical presentation, a diagnosis of enteric infection was considered and she was given intravenous antibiotics. Blood cultures drawn on admission were positive after 24 h incubation; the Gram stain showed poorly staining curved Gram-negative bacilli. The patient died the next day despite vigorous support in the Intensive Care Unit.

Questions

1. What is the likely diagnosis?
2. What are the other microbiological features of this organism?
3. What are the implications of this case for future travellers to Florida or similar environments?

Answers

1. The diagnosis is *Vibrio vulnificus* bacteraemia with septic shock in a patient with alcoholic liver disease. *Vibrio vulnificus* can cause wound infection or otitis externa following minor trauma sustained while swimming in salt waters at a high temperature as found in Florida and other American Gulf States. Such superficial infections may become rapidly cellu-

litic and necrotic and progress to septicaemia in persons with hepatic impairment. The case fatality from such septicaemia is 50–60% even when the diagnosis is considered early. Septicaemia can also arise in predisposed individuals following ingestion of contaminated seafood such as raw oysters and prawns. Empirical antimicrobial treatment for invasive disease should be intravenous tetracycline plus an aminoglycoside. Cefotaxime may be an alternative.

2. *Vibrio vulnificus* is one of the group of 'non-cholera' vibrios, so-called to distinguish them from classic cholera-producing *Vibrio cholerae*. Having said this, many of the group can cause severe toxin-mediated diarrhoeal disease. Many members can cause extra-intestinal disease including septicaemia and amongst these *Vibrio vulnificus* is the most virulent; the organism invades intestinal lymphatics to reach the bloodstream. It grows well on sheep blood agar producing pseudomonas-like large colonies which are oxidase positive. The Gram-stain shows curved Gram-negative bacilli suggestive of 'Vibrio' species. Species identification can be made using the API-20NE with the addition of 1% NaCl to the broth to aid growth; growth of vibrios of all species is enhanced by the addition of 1–2% NaCl.

3. All travellers to warm climates with known or potential chronic liver disease should be warned of the dangers of seabathing and ingestion of raw seafood.

Further reading

TACKET, C. O., BRENNER, F. and BLAKE, P. A. (1984) Clinical features and an epidemiologic study of *Vibrio vulnificus* infections. *J. Infect. Dis.*, **149**, 558.

Case 4   An elderly woman with abdominal pain and Gram-negative bacteraemia

A 90-year-old woman with a long history of rheumatoid arthritis who was maintained on steroid therapy fell and fractured her left humerus. Following internal fixation of the fracture, she was admitted to another hospital for rehabilitation. After 1 month in the second hospital she developed diarrhoea but was otherwise well. One week later, the diarrhoea worsened and was accompanied by abdominal pain and generalized tenderness. There was no guarding and bowel sounds were normal. At this time, her temperature was 38.4°C and she was transferred to an acute care hospital for rehydration and therapy of suspected intra-abdominal infection. On admission she was treated with cefuroxime and metronidazole. Blood cultures drawn prior to antimicrobial treatment were positive within 24 h for Gram-negative bacilli and cefuroxime was replaced by ciprofloxacin. Other investigations showed the following; WBC $6.3 \times 10^9/l$, Hb 11.6 g/dl, platelets $402 \times 10^9/l$. Na 124 mmol/l, K 4.1 mmol/l; LFTs, abdominal ultrasound and chest X-ray were all normal. The organism grew in both aerobic and anaerobic blood culture bottles and on sub-culture grew on blood agar aerobically and anaerobically, chocolate agar in CO_2 and MacConkey agar in air, all incubated at 35°C. The isolate was oxidase negative and Gram-staining showed short Gram-negative bacilli with a central area of pallor (bipolar staining). The abdominal pain at this stage became localized in the right iliac fossa.

Questions

1. What is the differential diagnosis?
2. How would you proceed to identify the organism further?
3. How was the organism likely to have been acquired and what do you know of its epidemiology?

Answers

1. The differential diagnosis in infection may change rapidly depending on the evolution of the disease process. Starting with the abdominal symptoms and signs and, the (presumably) associated bacteraemia, diagnoses would include surgical conditions such as diverticulitis or appendix abscess and exogenous enteric infections. In the former, bacteraemia would likely be with *E. coli* or *Bacteroides sp.* Exogenous causes, particularly causing bacteraemia in an elderly patient, include *Salmonella* sp., e.g. *S. typhimurium, Shigella, Campylobacter* and *Yersinia enterolitica*.
2. The growth features of the organism suggests a member of the enterobacteriaceae but bi-polar staining should raise the

particular possibility of *Yersinia*. Further identification should be attempted with the API 20E (as with other enterobacteriaeceae). The organism did in fact code on the API 20E as *Y. enterocolitica* and this was compatible with the clinical findings.

3. *Yersinia enterocolitica* is a member of the enterobacteriaceae. It shows frequent pleomorphism on Gram-staining and bipolar staining (as with other *Yersinia* spp.) *Yersinia* infections are apparently uncommon in the UK, although many laboratories do not routinely look for this organism in faeces. It is associated with the temperate climates of Europe and North America and this is probably because growth is optimal at 22–29°C. Isolation from faeces requires the use of the selective CIN medium (cefsulodin – irgasan – novobiocin) with incubation at room temperature. Recovery from blood and other sterile body fluids is good on routine media. Mesenteric adenitis and terminal ileitis are frequent presentations in older children and adults. Septicaemia occurs when there are predisposing conditions, which in this case were old age and steroid use. The organism is principally acquired from contaminated food, and several outbreaks have been described. Epidemiological investigations in this case implicated food brought into hospital by family members.

Further reading

MEGRAUD, F. (1987) *Yersinia* infection and acute abdominal pain. *Lancet*, **1**, 1147.

Case 5 A pelvic mass

A 35-year-old housewife was referred to the hospital with complaints of weight loss and weakness. Ten days earlier, she had noticed the onset of a yellowish vaginal discharge and lower abdominal pain for which the GP prescribed amoxycillin. On the day of admission she complained of pains in the upper abdomen and pelvis. She was nulligravida and had no history of sexually transmitted diseases, but was sexually active with an intrauterine device *in situ*.

On physical examination her temperature was 39°C, and the blood pressure was 150/70 mmHg. Examination of the chest and heart were normal. Examination of the abdomen showed tenderness in the left upper and lower quadrants and shotty inguinal lymph nodes. Pelvic examination showed bilateral adnexal fullness and a fluctuant mass extending from the left pelvis midway to the umbilicus. The external genitalia were normal.

Blood values were Hb 5.1g/dl, WBC 25.7×10^9/l, platelets 219×10^9/l. The albumin was 21 g/l but serum chemistry was otherwise normal. VDRL was negative, CEA, colloid antigen 125 and β-HCG were all normal. There were no Bence–Jones proteins in urine; HIV serology and tuberculin skin testing were negative. A chest X-ray was normal and blood cultures were negative. CT scan of the abdomen showed a large pelvic mass of mixed density.

Laparotomy was performed and large bilateral tubo-ovarian abscesses exuding frank pus were found; the uterus was of normal size. The patient underwent bilateral salpingo-oophorectomy with supracervical hysterectomy and excision involved segments of small and large bowel. A sinus track traversed the anterior peritoneum into the abdominal wall. Culture of samples obtained intraoperatively from the pelvic abscesses showed growth of *E. coli, Klebsiella pneumoniae, Bacteroides fragilis* and *Candida albicans*. She was treated with intravenous antibiotics and amphotericin post-operatively.

Questions

1. What was the likely underlying diagnosis which is *not* associated with sexual transmission?
2. How would you confirm your suspicions?

Answers

1. Pelvic actinomycosis associated with an IUD.
2. Microscopic examination of Fallopian tube sections to search for sulphur granules.

Comment

Actinomyces israelii is a saprophyte found commonly in the mouth and although the term 'myces' suggests that it is a fungus, it is actually a Gram-positive filamentous (higher) bacterium.

The Actinomyces are anaerobic, very slow growing, and they are also normal members of the vaginal flora. When they invade tissue, actinomyces tend to form 'sulphur granules' which can be seen with the naked eye. These granules are masses of mycelia cemented together by calcium phosphate, the result of the patient's own alkaline phosphatase activity. In the majority of cases with actinomycosis there is antecedent trauma (in this case with an IUD) and the infection is slowly progressive. Around half the infections are in the leg and neck area, 15% are in the chest and around 2% are abdominal. At all sites, the surrounding tissue shows chronic inflammation and fibrosis and direct extension through the skin can cause chronically draining sinuses, and in this case a sinus track was found. It has been recognized for over 20 years that heavy cervical colonization with actinomyces is a potential consequence of the use of an IUD and commonly this is asymptomatic. The reported prevalence of colonization by actinomyces in IUD users varies from 1.6–36%. However, some women using IUDs have been reported to suffer from invasive actinomycosis of the pelvis, bowel, liver, lung, heart, bladder and the brain.

Although the reasons for actinomyces colonization are not known, it has been suggested that breakdown of the endometrium by the IUD allows asymptomatic colonization to progress to infection. In most cases, removal of the IUD is sufficient, and antibiotics are not required.

Actinomyces organisms are difficult to culture, with yields as low as 4%. They must be cultured anaerobically and being equisitively sensitive to penicillin, such cultures will be negative if the patient has received penicillin prior to culture as in this case.

Blood cultures are rarely positive, and of course the growth of actinomyces from mouth swabs sputum or stool is not diagnostic. The main tests are culture of lesions, and Gram-staining of histological sections. Treatment is with excision and long-term penicillin therapy, intravenous for 3 months and oral for another 9 months. The outlook is very good, with only three reported deaths from pelvic actinomycosis.

Further reading

LESLIE, D. E. and GARLAND, S. M. (1991) Comparison of immunofluorescence and culture for the detection of *Actinomyces israelii* in wearers of intrauterine contraceptive devices. *J. Med. Microbiol.*, **35**, 224–228.

Case 6 Chronic fatigue with an acute swelling of the knee

A 55-year-old construction engineer had been in good health until 18 months previously when he returned from a summer holiday in Ontario, Canada. After his return, his wife had noticed a ring shaped red rash underneath his left armpit, followed some days later by other red circles on the body. He then developed headache, chills and a swelling of the left testicle. The rash and swelling subsided in a fortnight and he was left with a persistent feeling of fatigue. Two months later he was admitted to hospital as an emergency with neck stiffness, and lumbar puncture showed 100 lymphocytes/mm^3, protein 0.6 g/l and glucose 3.0 mm/dl. No treatment was given and he improved spontaneously. His present complaint was of pain and swelling in the right knee for 4 weeks. He was on extended sick leave from his job because of extreme fatigue but was learning to live with this. Further history in the outpatients clinic revealed that he had helped out on his brother's farm in Ontario, especially in the gardens. He had suffered many insect bites but could not recall a bite in the axilla.

On examination his was afebrile, pulse 80/min, BP 140/70 mmHg. There was no rash or lymphadenopathy and examination of the central nervous system, chest and abdomen were normal. The knee was swollen and an effusion was detected. Aspiration of the knee showed 25 000 neutrophils/mm^3, with no growth on culture. Full blood count and blood urea, electrolytes, liver function tests, immunoglobulin profile, antinuclear factor, rheumatoid factor, ESR and CRP were all normal and chest X-ray was clear. ECG was normal.

Questions

1. What is the probable diagnosis?
2. How effective is treatment likely to be?

Answers

1. Lyme disease.

2. 50% of cases of late onset arthritis complicating Lyme disease will be cured by antibiotics.

Comment

Lyme disease is caused by the spirochaete, *Borrelia burgdorferi*, and is transmitted by the bite of ixodid ticks, especially in the summer. As in other spirochaetal illnesses, there are many stages, which are demonstrative by this case.

Stage 1

After an incubation period of 3–32 days, a macule appears at the site of a bite and this expands to form the circular lesion as erythema migrans (EM; formerly erythema chronicum migrans). This is caused by the migration of spirochaetes through the skin and shows a central clearing. As in this case, most patients do not remember being bitten by a tick. The commonest sites for EM are the thigh, groin, and axilla. Following skin infection, spirochaetes enter the bloodstream producing further annular skin lesions at other sites. There is often severe headache, neck stiffness, fever, arthralgia and pronounced fatigue. Testicular swelling has been described in 1% of cases. Within several weeks, the first manifestations disappear, but persistent fatigue can be troublesome for many months.

Stage 2

Some months after stage 1, migrating pains can occur in tendons, muscles, joints and bone but there is no joint swelling. Around one-fifth of patients develop CNS complications, especially meningitis, facial nerve palsy or mononeuritis multiplex. A usual picture is of fluctuating meningitis with facial palsy. Examination of CSF reveals lymphocytes, elevated protein and normal glucose. These signs usually disappear within a few months. At this stage around 10% of patients can have cardiac disease, mainly various forms of heart block. Poor left ventricular function has been reported, often only lasting for a few weeks.

Stage 3

Up to 2 years after the original infection, 60% of patients develop a true arthritis most commonly affecting the large joints. Some patients have a symmetrical polyarthritis but the commonest presentation is swelling of one knee. By the stage of true arthritis, only fatigue remains of the systemic symptoms and the ESR and the immunoglobulin profiles which may have been abnormal early in the illness have returned to normal. Also, there is no fever. Attacks of arthritis can last around 6 weeks, resolve and recur numerous times over several years. The joint aspirate reveals high neutrophil counts, and the rheumatoid and antinuclear factors are negative.

The cause of this late disease appears to be persistence of the organism in synovial tissue, but attempts to culture the organism or visualize it directly are often unrewarding. The most useful laboratory test is the detection of specific IgG antibody to *B. burgdorferi*, which is virtually always present by the stage of arthritis, and in fact is often present after the first few weeks of the original illness. The treatment of Lyme disease depends on the stage of illness. Early disease is best treated with tetracycline 250 mg qds; and phenoxymethylpenicillin or erythromycin can also be used. Initially treatment is for 10 days, extending to 2 weeks if symptoms still persist. Following treatment, around 15% of patients develop a Jarisch–Herxheimer reaction manifested by sudden onset of fever (characteristically to 38.5°C), muscle pains, headache, and hypertension. There is tachycardia, tachypnoea and a moderate rise in the white cell count. The reaction lasts around 24 h and is treated with bed rest and aspirin. This reaction is also seen in other spirochaetal diseases such as syphilis and relapsing fever. In louse-borne relapsing fever this may be so severe as to cause death. In the case of late onset joint disease, a suitable treatment would be penicillin G in divided doses for 20 days. This is curative in around 50% of cases, and should this fail, surgical removal of the synovial tissue should be considered.

A more frequent 'rheumatological' problem in infectious diseases is that of a polyarthritis accompanied by fever. Table 1 shows the usual causes of this problem.

Table 1: Causes of fever and polyarthritis

Infections (bacteria, fungi, mycobacterial viral)
Post-infectious (gastrointestinal infections, genitourinary infection, rheumatic fever)
Rheumatoid arthritis and adult Still's disease
Connective tissues diseases (SLE, vasculitis)
Crystal deposition (gout, pseudogout)
Other (Mediterranean fever, sarcoid)

The highest priority should be given to synovial fluid microscopy and culture, as well as blood culture. Bacteria or crystals may be seen by microscopy and synovial white cell count in bacterial infections is frequently over 50 000/mm^3. If cultures of synovial fluid are unhelpful, then viral and atypical titres should be performed to include for post-infectious causes. Antinuclear factor, rheumatoid factor, and ASO titres should be measured, as well as the VDRL. The ESR is fairly non-diagnostic, as it is virtually always raised in the clinical situation of fever and polyarthritis. Rheumatoid arthritis should only be diagnosed as a matter of exclusion, and then only after some time has elapsed to observe the pattern of disease.

Further reading

JACOBS, J. C., STEVENS, M. AND DURAY, P.H. (1986) Lyme disease simulating septic arthritis. *JAMA*, **256**, 1138.

Case 7 An elderly woman with headache and vomiting

An 85-year-old female patient was admitted to hospital with increasing drowsiness, headache and vomiting. Admission findings included blood pressure 110/70 mmHg, heart rate 92/min, temperature 38.4°C and respiratory rate 22/min. On examination she appeared to be quite drowsy and was photophobic. A lumbar puncture performed after CT scanning showed 20 000 white cells per mm^3, 95% polymorphs. No organisms were seen on Gram-stain. Latex agglutination tests for *Neisseria meningitidis*, *Streptococcus pneumoniae* and *Haemophilus influenzae* antigens were negative. She was started on cefotaxime and penicillin with a presumptive diagnosis of pyogenic meningitis. The following day her cerebrospinal fluid culture was positive for a Gram-negative bacillus growing on blood agar, chocolate and MacConkey plates.

Questions

1. What organisms would you consider in the differential diagnosis of such pyogenic meningitis prior to the culture result?
2. What single critical test would you expect the laboratory to perform having established that the organism is Gram-negative and grows on blood, chocolate and MacConkey plates?
3. Should therapy be changed and for how long would you treat?

Answers

1. Possible organisms include the standard causes associated with adult meningitis such as *Neisseria meningitidis* and *Streptococcus pneumoniae*. *Haemophilus influenzae* would be extremely unusual in this age group, since after the age of 20 years most adults have antibodies to type b, the serotype associated with invasive disease. Organisms typically associated with neonatal meningitis tend to recur in this older age group, including *Listeria monocytogenes* and members of the enterobacteriaceae such as *E. coli, Klebsiella* etc. The possibility of infection with *P. aeruginosa* should be considered because this organism is occasionally not covered by standard empirical antimicrobial regimens and together with *E. coli* and *Klebsiella*, accounts for the majority of Gram-negative bacillary meningitis. Fungal meningitis caused by *Cryptococcus neoformans* is uncommon in the non-immuno-compromised host; however, it does occur, particularly when there is a convergence of risk factors, such as old age and steroid therapy. If cryptococcal meningitis is suspected because of risk factors (or failure of clinical response), then latex agglutination tests for cryptococcal polysaccharide antigen should be done on the CSF sample. The India ink test is neither specific nor sensitive and its use is to be discouraged. Both fungal meningitis and tuberculous meningitis would be expected to present with lymphocytic pictures in the CSF as would an acute viral meningitis.
2. The most helpful test having determined that a bacterium is Gram-negative and non-fastidious (grows on blood, chocolate and MacConkey plates), is the oxidase test. This test differentiates members of the enterobacteriaceae such as *E. coli, Klebsiella, Enterobacter* etc., from pseudomonas species and in particular *P. aeruginosa* (oxidase positive).

3. The optimal therapy for Gram-negative bacillary meningitis caused by *E. coli*, *Klebsiella*, other enterobacteriaceae or *P. aeruginosa* is unknown. This issue is of increasing importance as the number of such cases continues to rise, most commonly associated with head trauma, neurosurgery or Gram-negative bacteraemia from an extracranial primary site. Since most cases are associated with hospital-acquired flora, local patterns of resistance must be taken into account in the choice of empirical therapy, and laboratory data on any isolate carefully examined. Most authorities would recommend a third generation cephalosporin in high doses as empirical therapy, because of broad spectrum cover and high drug levels in the CSF. Cefotaxime is therefore a good choice, but it must be remembered that of the common third generation agents only ceftazidime additionally covers *P. aeruginosa*. Although aminoglycoside levels in the CSF are relatively low, one of these agents is frequently added in confirmed cases for optimal therapy of the frequently associated Gram-negative bacteraemia and the primary focus of dissemination. In the face of clinical failure and/or evidence of emergence of drug resistance to a third generation cephalosporin on therapy, an Ommaya or Rickman reservoir is frequently placed for intraventricular aminoglycoside administration together with systemic aminoglycoside, and an 'anti-pseudomonal' penicillin such as piperacillin. Some authorities advocate this line whenever *P. aeruginosa* is the pathogen involved. Note also that penicillin is still the drug of choice for *N. meningitidis* and sensitive *S. pneumoniae* so that the initial choice of penicillin + cefotaxime was reasonable (with the caveat that cefotaxime does not cover *P. aeruginosa*). It is also important to note that in the post-neurosurgical patient, *S. aureus* comes into the differential diagnosis and flucloxacillin should be added. Optimal *empirical* cover in the post-neurosurgical patient might therefore be: ceftazidime + gentamicin + flucloxacillin.

Further reading

ANDERSON, M. (1993) Management of cerebral infection. *Journal of Neurology, Neurosurgery, and Psychiatry*, **56**, 1243–1258.

Case 8   Yeasts in one blood culture bottle

A 72-year-old man underwent open heart surgery for replacement of a stenosed aortic valve. The operation was performed with flucloxacillin and gentamicin administered as prophylaxis for post-operative wound infection. This regimen was continued for 1 week when it was replaced by teicoplanin and ceftazidime for suspected sepsis. Blood cultures drawn from central lines and peripheral veins were positive in multiple bottles for coagulase - negative staphylococci and all lines were changed. The ceftazidime was continued along with teicoplanin because of heavy growth of *P. aeruginosa* from endotracheal secretions. After $2\frac{1}{2}$ weeks the patient was still ventilated, on teicoplanin and ceftazidime, and then developed another episode of 'sepsis'. The sternotomy wound was healing well and there was no obvious focus of infection. Blood cultures grew a yeast in one out of four bottles (1/2, 0/2) from two sets; Gram stain of the broth suggested *Candida* sp. Empirical therapy was begun with fluconazole.

Questions

1. Is this disseminated candidiasis?
2. What are the possible risk factors for candida fungaemia?
3. What is the likelihood of candidal endocarditis developing?
4. Was the empirical treatment of the yeast appropriate?

Answers

1. The finding of yeasts in a blood culture should always be considered significant until proven otherwise and particularly in anatomically or immunologically compromised patients. *Candida* sp. causing fungaemia are increasing as invasive medical technology advances and with more immune-compromised patients in hospital. At the stage of the history given, all that can be said is that the patient has apparent fungaemia with yeasts likely to be *Candida* sp. Germ tube

positivity will distinguish albicans from non-albicans candida. Whilst disseminated candidiasis is possible, such a diagnosis requires evidence of multi-organ involvement.
2. Risk factors predisposing to candidaemia are three-fold:

   (i) alteration of normal flora by broad spectrum antibacterial agents or combinations leading to candida overgrowth, particularly in the bowel.
   (ii) disruption of anatomical barriers to infection such as with central vascular lines.
   (iii) compromised immune status as in chemotherapy induced neutropenia.
   Items (i) and (ii) were certainly applicable to this patient. The prophylactic regimen was continued for far too long a period; most authorities would cover for no more than 24 h. Treating the *P. aeruginosa* should have been based on more evidence of infection as opposed to just colonization.

3. The most likely source of candida in this patient is a central vascular line. If all lines are removed or changed, then with appropriate antifungal agents it is unlikely that endocarditis will develop. The longer the period of fungaemia, the greater the likelihood of seeding the valvular prosthesis and other distant sites, hence the need for a high index of suspicion and early treatment.
4. In the setting described it was appropriate that antifungal therapy was started, though most authorities would begin with amphotericin B pending identification of the isolate as albicans or otherwise. *Candida krusei*, for example, is inherently resistant to fluconazole. Note that blood culture systems for recovery of candida are sub-optimal and fungaemia may be present with negative blood cultures. A positive culture (even one bottle) must be considered to be significant unless it can be proven otherwise.

Further reading

BODEY, G. P. (1988) The emergence of fungi as major hospital pathogens. *J. Hosp. Infect.*, **11** (Suppl. A), 411–426.

Case 9 An archaeology student with haemoptysis

A 24-year-old archaeology student was admitted to hospital for investigation of haemoptysis. He began to feel unwell 5 months earlier, when he had noticed night sweats, tiredness and developed a cough eventually productive of blood. He was treated with antibiotics by his GP, following which the night sweats stopped and the haemoptysis lessened. The GP had sent sputum for microscopy including acid-fast bacilli and bacterial culture which had both been negative. His present admission to hospital was precipitated by a severe bout of haemoptysis. The patient was British and had an unremarkable previous medical history except that at the age of 20 he had suffered an episode of 'bronchitis' in Mexico whilst working on an archaeological dig. He had spent a total of 6 months in that country and admitted to having eaten pickled freshwater crabs whilst he was over there but had not become ill as a consequence. He was a non-smoker, heterosexual and drank very little alcohol. His weight was steady, and exercise tolerance normal. He kept no pets.

On examination he looked well: temperature 37.1°C, pulse 60/min, respiratory rate 18/min, BP was 110/60 mmHg, and no lymphadenopathy was found. He was not clubbed. There were diminished breath sounds over the left upper lobe but examination was otherwise entirely normal. Urine analysis was normal by dipstick testing. Laboratory investigations showed: Hb 14.0 g/dl; WBC 7.8×10^9/l (normal differential), platelets 189×10^9/l, urea and electrolytes, liver enzymes and clotting screen normal; Legionella antibodies were negative. A chest X-ray was reported as: 'there is a cavitating lesion with an airfluid level in the left upper lobe and consolidation in the left lower lobe'; a CT scan of the thorax was reported: there is a thin walled cavity in the left upper lobe (2.5 cm diameter) and left lower lobe consolidation. No lymphadenopathy seen. No pleural effusion is present'. FEV1, FVC and KCO were normal and sputum microscopy was reported 'a few white cells, no fungi or AFB'. Mycobacterial cultures of sputum requested by the GP 8 weeks earlier were still negative. Bronchoscopy showed blood in all segments, more so on the left. There were no endobronchial lesions. Bronchoalveolar lavage showed no malignant cells, acid-fast bacilli, fungi, ova or parasites.

Further negative investigations were glomerular basement membrane antibody, antineutrophil cytoplasmic antibody (ANCA), HIV antibodies and tuberculin skin test.

The temperature became normal without treatment in hospital and a further chest X-ray a week later showed that the fluid level in the cavity had disappeared.

Questions

1. What is the likely diagnosis?
2. What would you discuss with the patient as the next consideration for treatment?

Answers

1. Previous coccidioidomycosis with bleeding into the old cavity.
2. Wedge resection of the lesion from the left upper lobe.

Comment

This patient has a fluid filled cavity in the left upper lobe and on bronchoscopy the fluid was found to be blood. The consolidation reported in the left lower lobe was probably also produced by blood overflowing from the cavity.

The differential diagnosis of a cavitating lesion would include:
1. Necrotizing infection with bacteria (*Staph. aureus*, Klebsiella, Nocardia), mycobacteria (tuberculosis and atypical), fungi (Histoplasma, Aspergillus, Coccidioides) and parasites (amoebic abscess).
2. Pulmonary infarction (embolism or vasculitis).
3. Malignancy (primary or metastatic carcinoma).
4. Miscellaneous lesions such as infected cysts, silicosis and coal miner's pneumoconiosis.

The first practical consideration should be TB, for clinical and public health reasons. However, in this case, staining of broncho-alveolar lavage fluid was negative. A cavitating lesion due to TB is usually teeming with acid-fast bacilli and the tuberculin test was also negative.

The most striking feature of the X-ray was a *thin walled* cyst, which would make malignancy and Wegener's granulomatosis unlikely as these produce thick walled cavities. Goodpasture's syndrome does not produce cavities but rather diffuse alveolar haemorrhage.

His work in Mexico and the non-specific chest infection caused there should expand the differential diagnosis. Paragonimiasis occurs in Northern South America. Clinically this presents as chronic bronchitis and haemoptysis and chest X-rays show diffuse infiltrates in the lower and mid-lung fields, gradually replaced by round 3 cm nodules which not infrequently cavitate. However, in this case there was no eosinophilia and no ova were found in the sputum.

Another disease to consider is melioidosis. This is produced by the Gram-negative bacillus, *Burkholderia* (*Pseudomonas*) *pseudomallei* but this has only very rarely been described outside South East Asia, in Panama and Equador. This produces thin walled cavities around 5 cm in diameter and infection may present or be reactivated up to 20 years following acute exposure. In this case, microscopic examination of sputum did not reveal the characteristic small Gram-negative bacilli and they usually grow well on most laboratory media. The picture is not that of chronic histoplasmosis which mainly occurs in those over 40 years, and virtually always in smokers. Chronic histoplasmosis has an onset over weeks, with weight loss and bilateral apical infiltrates on chest X-ray. Chronic histoplasmosis eventually produces cavitation and retraction of both upper lobes.

In this case, it is probable that he had had an acute infection with the fungus *Coccidioides immitis* whilst working in dusty conditions in Mexico as part of his study. This is a soil saprophyte found in California, Arizona and Central America and infection follows inhalation. Only 40% of individuals develop symptoms, most of which are self-limiting after an incubation period of around 2 weeks. Usually a primary pulmonary infection will heal completely or less commonly leave a single thin walled cavity as in this case. A chest X-ray during his original illness in Mexico might have shown an infiltrate, hilar lymphadenopathy or pleural effusion, and blood counts would have shown a mild eosinophilia.

Serology can be helpful in coccidiomycosis, especially in disseminated disease, but can be misleading in the case of a solitary pulmonary cavity. Chest infection with *C. immitis* can be progressive, with cough, fever and weight loss, and may become disseminated. Treatment is with Amphotericin B or an anti-fungal azole.

Primary pulmonary disease is usually left untreated as it normally resolves.

Thin walled cavities tend to close spontaneously and are not normally resected but in this case the patient developed bacterial superinfection which caused haemorrhage into the cavity.

Further reading

DRUTZ, D. (1983) Amphotericin B in the treatment of coccidioidomycosis. *Drugs*, **26**, 337.

DRUTZ, D. J. and HUPPERT, M. (1983) Coccidioidomycosis: factors affecting the host-parasite interaction. *J. Infect. Dis.*, **147**: 372.

Case 10 Acute neurological deterioration in a Somalian student

A 35-year-old student of economics had been at university in the UK for 2 years. His home was in Somalia, which he had visited several times since the start of his studies.

He went to see his general practitioner because he felt generally unwell and had lost his appetite. Routine blood tests were performed in the surgery, showing Hb 13.4 g/dl, WBC 3.0×10^9/l, platelets 100×10^9/l, ESR 70 mm/h, urea and electrolytes normal. The bilirubin was 30 μmol/l, AST 60 IU/l and alkaline phosphatase 180 IU/l. As the patient had returned from Somalia 10 days previously, the general practitioner requested thick and thin blood films for malaria which were negative.

The following day the patient developed pain in the left iliac fossa and diarrhoea, and he was admitted to hospital.

He was married with two children still in Somalia. He did not drink or smoke and did not eat pork. On first arriving in the UK routine stool microscopy had shown *Giardia lamblia*, ascaris and *E. histolytica* and he had received treatment with metronidazole. A chest X-ray at that point had been normal.

Examination showed a temperature of 39.5°C, pulse 110/min, BP 110/70 mmHg. He looked unwell and slightly jaundiced, but no rash was seen. The lungs were clear and there was a grade 1 systolic murmur in the heart, and the tip of the spleen could just be felt. There was no hepatomegaly and neurological examination was negative apart from some drowsiness and confusion about the date. There was no neck stiffness or papilloedema.

Laboratory investigations showed Hb 11.2 g/dl, WBC 3.2×10^9/l, platelets 80×10^9/l, sodium 142 mmol/l, potassium 3.6 mmol/l, urea 8 mmol/l, creatinine 200 μmol/l. A chest X-ray was clear and an ECG was normal. Stool cultures sent by the general practitioner 24 h previously were still negative. Whilst he was being investigated he was found to be unrousable by the nurses and examination showed decorticate posturing and extensor plantar response.

Questions

1. What are the two urgent blood results required?
2. What potentially fatal respiratory complication may occur in 4 days time?

Answers

1. Thick films for malarial parasites and blood glucose.
2. Acute pulmonary oedema.

Comment

This patient is pyrexial with a rapidly developing anaemia, thrombocytopenia and neurological deterioration. He had returned from Africa 10 days prior to his presentation and so falciparum malaria *must* be suspected (see Table 1 for complications of falciparum malaria). Approximately ten patients die in the United Kingdom each year from falciparum malaria, and the commonest error is to ascribe the symptoms to flu. Many immigrants to the United Kingdom believe they have a natural immunity to malaria and do not take prophylaxis when visiting their families abroad. One-third of falciparum malaria cases occur in this group. The presentation of falciparum malaria may be very non-specific, with a cough, abdominal pain, diarrhoea or muscle aches. Fever is usual, but of course there can be periods when the patient will be afebrile. In any type of malaria, splenomegaly is found in less than half the patients and should not be relied on as a sign.

In this case, that of cerebral malaria, the rapid progression of falciparum malaria is demonstrated. For diagnosing malaria, a thick film is much more sensitive than a thin film and negative films do not exclude the diagnosis. A thorough evaluation should involve examination of blood smears every 8 h over a period of 3 days if the diagnosis is suspected. In this case, only one film had been sent. Falciparum malaria is described as 'severe' if the level of parasitaemia is 2% or above or if the patient cannot take oral fluid. However, even if the initial parasitaemia is very low as in this case, the course of the disease can be fulminant over a few days.

Table 1 Complications of falciparum malaria

Cerebral malaria
Renal failure
Shock
Profound anaemia
Disseminated intravascular coagulation
Pulmonary oedema

Cerebral malaria occurs when the microcirculation of the brain is occluded because of adhesion of parasitized red cells to capillaries and post-capillary venules. This produces an encephalopathy manifested by convulsions, extensor posturing, general flaccidity, or irregular breathing. The blood sugar must be measured every 4 h because hypoglycaemia can complicate falciparum malaria and present with exactly the same features as cerebral malaria. Hypoglycaemia can also occur as a side effect of quinine treatment, so monitoring of the glucose levels must be kept up for a prolonged period. Other causes of neurological deterioration in falciparum malaria apart from cerebral malaria are electrolyte disturbances, anaemia and hypoxia and these should also be sought.

Renal failure can also occur and this should be treated with intravenous fluid, diuretics and renal doses of dopamine. It is vital that the fluid input should be guided by measurement of the central venous pressure, or if at all possible, pulmonary artery wedge pressure. Myocardial function is usually well preserved but pulmonary oedema can be produced by leakage out of capillaries producing a picture similar to the adult respiratory distress syndrome. Artificial ventilation may be required in these cases and the mortality of this complication is 80%.

The treatment of falciparum malaria is usually with oral quinine sulphate 600 mg tds for 7 days. Three Fansidar tablets are also usually given. By definition, in severe malaria intravenous quinine is required with each dose being infused slowly over 4 h. Oral therapy should be commenced as soon as the patient is able to swallow.

In an immigrant from a tropical country, loss of consciousness should still be investigated by CT head scan and lumbar puncture even if malaria parasites are found in the blood. This is because conditions like bacterial meningitis would be missed in the presence of coincidental malarial infestation.

General management includes keeping the temperature below 38.5°C by sponging and paracetamol but treatment of cerebral malaria with dexamethasone or mannitol should be avoided. In the past, both heparin and steroids were given in cerebral malaria, which lead to a high incidence of gastrointestinal bleeding. It is usual to monitor the parasitaemia twice a day until the films become negative, and they should be repeated if fever recurs. Transfusion of fresh blood should be given if the Hb falls below 8 g/dl and regular blood cultures should be performed.

Patients presenting with a fever after return from the tropics should be suspected of having malaria or typhoid until proven otherwise. Most tropical diseases can be diagnosed by full blood count (with malaria screen), stool culture and microscopy, blood culture, hepatitis serology, viral and atypical serology including Q fever and chlamydia and an arbovirus virus screen suitable to the location of travel. Urine culture and microscopy, and a chest X-ray to screen for TB should also be performed. If the fever is prolonged, then ultrasound of the abdomen may be useful to detect an amoebic liver abscess, assess the size of the spleen and search for pyogenic foci.

Further reading

WHITE, N. J., WARRELL, D. A., CHANTAVANICH, P. et al (1983) Severe hypoglycaemia and hyperinsulinaemia in falciparum malaria. N. Engl. J. Med., **309**, 61–66.
WYLER, D. J. (1988) Steroids are out in the treatment of cerebral malaria: what's next? J. Infect. Dis., **158**, 320–324.

Case 11   Dysphagia following a nail puncture

A 4-year-old boy from an Irish gypsy family now living in Britain sustained a puncture wound to his right heel from a rusty nail whilst playing barefoot near his parents' caravan site. The lesion was apparently quite small with no visible bleeding and no first aid was given. Some 10 days later he began to complain of vague pain at the site of the puncture. Two days later he complained of difficulty in swallowing and pain in the neck aggravated by movement. He was taken to the admissions unit of the local hospital in quite an irritable state. On admission, the child was crying, in considerable distress and holding the neck area.

Questions

1. What is the likely diagnosis?
2. What is the management?
3. What is the prognosis?

Answers

1. The history and presentation is typical of tetanus, a very uncommon disease in developed countries because of successful immunization programmes. This child had only received one dose of vaccine to date because of the travelling lifestyle. The spores of the causative anaerobe, *Clostridium tetani*, are so ubiquitous that the incidence and mortality of tetanus are high where immunization programmes are not developed. For the same reason, growth of *C. tetani* from superficial swabs in no way establishes a diagnosis of tetanus; the diagnosis is clinical and must be immediate. The neurotoxin from *C. tetani*, tetanospasmin, blocks the release of inhibitory neurotransmitters and so promotes unrestrained firing of motor neurones to opposing muscle groups, resulting in painful contraction and muscular spasm.
2. The patient should be admitted to the Intensive Care Unit because of the need for sedation (with a benzodiazepine) and possible therapeutic paralysis to control severe muscle spasms. Human tetanus immunoglobulin should be administered to bind unbound tetanospasmin. Penicillin G is given to

decrease and ultimately stop the replication of the organism and hence further toxin production. Oral metronidazole has also been used.

3. This child responded very well to the measures outlined and did not require ventilation, but the overall mortality rate for generalized tetanus is around 25–30% even with optimal care. Poor prognostic features include; an incubation period of less than 9 days, onset of generalized spasms within 48 h of the first symptoms, severe generalized tetanus, and secondary (nosocomial) pneumonia.

Comment

The spores of *C. tetani* are extremely stable in the environment and can cause disease in any non-immune person. In developing countries, failure of immunization programmes is the major cause of this preventable disease. With an incomplete course of vaccinations, the child in this case was susceptible; however, partial immunity may have decreased the severity of the illness. Routine booster injections are indicated every 10 years after a full primary course.

Strychnine poisoning and dystonic reactions from dopaminergic antagonists also come into the differential diagnosis of tetanus but the history and presentation in this case are diagnostic.

Further reading

OLSEN, K.M. and HILLER, F.C. (1987) Management of tetanus. *Clin. Pharm.*, **6**, 570.

Case 12   Necrotizing lymphadenitis in a child

A 6-year-old girl was referred to the infectious diseases clinic a week after the sudden onset of fever, poor appetite and lethargy. Examination showed a tender lymph node in the right axilla and a papule on the dorsum of the right hand, 2 mm in diameter. Examination of the nervous system was normal; the chest was clear but the tip of the spleen was palpable 2 cm below the costal margin.

One week after her appointment, the patient developed a fever of 40°C, and suffered sudden loss of vision in the right eye. She was seen again at the clinic and visual acuity was reduced to counting fingers with the right eye and normal with the left. Fundoscopy showed optic disc swelling and a retinal detachment on the right side. Again a tender lymph node (1 cm diameter) was felt in the right axilla and the spleen was still palpable.

Blood tests showed Hb 12.5 g/dl, WBC 5.6×10^9/l (17% atypical lymphocytes, 2% eosinophils), platelets 346×10^9/l. The ESR was 40 mm/h, and the monospot test was negative. VDRL, ASO, hepatitis B surface antigen, CMV IgG and HIV antibody tests were all negative. Liver function tests and angiotensin converting enzyme level were normal. Epstein–Barr virus serology was negative as was toxocara serology. Blood cultures were negative.

Lumbar puncture showed 61 WBC per mm^3 (99% mononuclear cells) and three red blood cells; total protein was 20 mg/l, glucose 3 mmol/l. No organisms were seen. Abdominal ultrasound showed hepatosplenomegaly with no focal lesions. Bacterial and viral cultures of CSF and urine were negative. The patient was treated with pyrimethamine, sulphadiazine and folinic acid for suspected toxoplasmosis. However, toxoplasma IgG and IgM serology proved to be negative and therefore the axilliary node was excised. Gram stain of the node showed no organisms and aerobic, anaerobic, mycobacterial, fungal and viral cultures of the node were negative. Histologically, the lymph node showed necrotizing granulomatous lymphadenitis with multiple micro-abscesses. Methylene and Giemsa's stains were negative. Further history indicated that the family cat had given birth to a litter of kittens and the girl had been scratched several times over the previous few months. Her brother of 8 and a sister of 4 years were also reported to have had scratches on their hands and painful swellings under their armpits. You are called to give your opinion of this case.

Questions

1. What is the likely diagnosis?
2. What treatment would you suggest?

Answers

1. Cat-scratch disease. (CSD)

2. Intravenous dexamethasone 1.2 mg/kg/day and i.v. co-trimoxazole 10 mg/kg/day.

Comment

Cat-scratch disease is characterized by enlargement of a regional lymph node following a scratch, bite or lick from a cat. Occasionally the disease presents with conjunctivitis and preauricular lymphadenopathy, and this is known as Parinaud's oculoglandular syndrome.

Cat-scratch disease occurs throughout the world, and 75% of patients will give a history of cat contact. The animal is usually a kitten and family outbreaks can occur and, as in this case, the infected cats are quite healthy. Patients appear generally well, and 50% have involvement of a single lymph node, the enlargement usually persisting for 3 months. Although most patients suffer a mild illness, encephalitis and radiculitis, or as in this case, neuroretinitis can occur. Patients with CNS involvement experience sudden onset of neurological deficit along with fever around 2 weeks after the onset of lymphadenopathy. The CSF is usually normal but there may be a mild elevation of protein.

The diagnosis of cat scratch disease is in many cases clinical and is suggested in this case by slowly developing lymphadenopathy, a history of cat scratches with the papule (inoculation site) and the histology of the excised node. Tenderness of the lymph node suggests an inflammatory process such as 'bacterial' adenitis caused by *S. aureus, S. pyogenes* or, cat-scratch disease rather than a tumour.

The cat scratch antigen skin test is positive in 90% of the patients clinically suspected of having cat scratch disease. However, a positive test may not reflect active disease, but merely exposure. The antigen is made from pus aspirated from a human sufferer's lymph node and because it is only heated to 56°C, the possibility of transmitting infectious agents makes it a test of last resort. In this case staining of the node with a Warthin Starry silver stain was positive for 'cat scratch bacilli'.

Most evidence points to *Bartonella henselae* (formerly Rochalimaea) as the major cause of cat scratch disease. It is found in 84% of patients with suspected cat scratch disease compared to 3.6% of healthy controls. The organism has been found in lymph nodes by culture, polymerase chain reaction and immunocytochemistry. Serologic evidence of infection can be obtained by an IFA assay where a titre of >1:64 is considered positive.

There are no controlled trials of treatment for this syndrome, but *in vitro* activity against the bacillus has been shown with cefotaxime, ciprofloxacin, co-trimoxazole, rifampicin and gentamicin. In CNS involvement, gentamicin should not be used as its penetration into CSF is poor.

The majority of patients with cat scratch disease recover without any treatment.

The condition, Leber's idiopathic stellate neuroretinitis, presents with unilateral macular exudates and papillitis which resolve spontaneously in around 2 months with no serious sequelae, and a few of these cases have been associated with cat scratch exposures. It may be that this is yet another form of cat scratch disease.

Further reading

CARITHERS, H. A. (1985) Cat-scratch disease: an overview based on 1200 patients. *Am. J. Dis. Child.*, **139**, 1124.

Case 13   Otitis externa in a diabetic patient

A 65-year-old male insulin-dependent diabetic patient presented to an emergency department with a painful swelling of his right ear which had developed acutely over the previous 36 h. On examination the pinna was hot, red and tender with swelling and erythema extending into the adjacent soft tissues. There was a serous discharge from the external auditory meatus. The patient appeared to be systemically unwell with a temperature of 38.4°C, heart rate of 86 per minute and he was sweating. He was an avid swimmer and had suffered episodes of otitis externa in the past which responded to local therapy.

Questions

1. What is the most serious potential diagnosis?
2. What is the immediate management?

Answers

1. The most serious potential diagnosis is that this is so called 'malignant' otitis externa which is principally caused by *Pseudomonas aeruginosa*. The process is necrotising and spreads from superficial tissues to involve adjacent structures including cartilage, nerve fibres, blood vessels and bone. It is particularly associated with diabetes mellitus but must be considered in any compromised patient. Deeper tissue involvement is both a medical and surgical emergency with possible bacteraemia, meningitis, brain abscess and venous thrombosis. Whilst CT and MRI scanning can assist in determining the extent of spread, a high index of suspicion of such spread and immediate clinical evaluation, including surgical consultation, are vital in this life threatening condition. Clinical findings include otalgia, hearing loss, local tenderness, skin discoloration and a discharge from the external auditory meatus. Signs of systemic toxicity may or may not be present depending upon the degree of invasion.

2. The patient should be given systemic antimicrobial therapy immediately with optimal cover for *P. aeruginosa*, including beta-lactam - aminoglycoside combinations, e.g. ceftazidime plus gentamicin, depending on prevailing resistance patterns. Depending on the extent of tissue necrosis, medical therapy only will fail unless dead/devitalized tissue is surgically removed. Systemic antimicrobials are given for 4–6 weeks. Oral ciprofloxacin has been used successfully when employed early in the course of this disease. Remember to submit surgically removed tissue for microbiological examination – swabs from the external auditory canal are not a substitute!

Further reading

LANG, R., GOSHAN, S., KITZES-COHEN, R. *et al.* (1990) Successful treatment of malignant external otitis with oral ciprofloxacin: Report of experience with 23 patients. *J. Infect. Dis.*, **161**, 537.

GIAMARELLOU, H. (1992) Malignant otitis externa: the therapeutic evolution of a lethal infection. *J. Antimicrob. Chemother.*, **30**, 745–751.

Case 14   Fever on return from Sierra Leone

A 25-year-old British doctor left his job as a gastroenterology registrar at a British hospital to do voluntary work for a year in Eastern Sierra Leone. He had come back to visit his parents and been well for the first 2 weeks, but then consulted his general practitioner with malaise. The next day, he reported that every muscle in his body was painful, especially his back. He was given some antibiotics but on the third day of illness he developed a cough, and on the fourth day a sore throat. He also had epigastric pain made worse on sitting forward and a separate lower abdominal pain. He was clearly deteriorating and on the seventh day of illness he was confined to bed with vomiting and diarrhoea. He called his general practitioner to see him at home and from there he was admitted to the hospital.

On examination he looked very anxious and sweaty, and appeared very unwell. Temperature was 38°C, BP 100/70 mmHg, pulse 97/min, respiratory rate 23/min. Examination of the throat showed an exudative pharyngitis and examination of the chest revealed a pericardial friction rub and dullness to percussion and reduced breath sounds at the left lung base. Abdominal examination was normal. Nervous system examination was normal apart from generalized weakness. A blood film for malaria was negative and chest X-ray showed a small left pleural effusion.

During the next day he became breathless, confused and had some swelling of the face. There was no skin rash and the blood pressure fell to 80 by palpation.

Examination of the blood showed Hb 10.7 g/dl, WBC 5.9×10^9/l, platelets 305×10^9l, clotting screen normal. Sodium 136 mmol/l, potassium 5.0 mmol/l, urea 27 mmol/l, AST 408 IU/l, alkaline phosphatase normal. Creatine phosphokinase was 515 IU/l and dipstick testing of the urine was positive for protein.

Questions

1. What is the diagnosis?
2. What is the most useful treatment that you can give him?

Answers

1. Lassa fever.

2. Ribavirin.

This is a classical presentation of Lassa fever. Each Health Authority will have its own plan regarding the management of viral haemorrhagic fevers, and this should be read in good time rather than on the night of admission of a suspected case.

Comment

Lassa virus is a member of the Arena virus family, and the disease is named after a town in Nigeria where a missionary nurse was infected in 1969. Since that time, outbreaks have been recognised in Northern Nigeria, Liberia and Eastern Sierra Leone. In Sierra Leone, the disease is endemic with half the elderly population possessing antibodies against Lassa fever virus. In Eastern Sierra Leone, 30% of all adult medical deaths are due to Lassa fever and Lassa fever accounts for 10% of hospital admissions presenting with pyrexia. However, it is now known that many cases are sub-clinical and the overall fatality rate much lower than previously thought. The persons most at risk of infection are hospital staff in these countries, and 10% of hospital personnel in Liberia have Lassa fever antibodies.

The animal reservoir of infection is a common rat. Surveys in Sierra Leone show that there is around one rat per household, and many of these rats excrete the virus in urine. Transmission between humans can occur by urine, faeces, saliva and accidental inoculation during hospital procedures. The incubation period is at most 24 days and therefore a patient presenting after that period outside West Africa can be considered not to have Lassa fever. All patients who are infected have a fever and malaise, and around half have headaches and half the patients will have muscle pain. Four days into the illness the patient might seek medical advice, by which time he is vomiting and experiencing chest, abdominal and back pains. An early symptom is pharyngitis and after a week white exudates or ulcers may be seen in the mouth. The patient may have generalized painless lymphadenopathy and a pericarditis and pleural effusion are extremely suggestive of Lassa fever. In fact, Lassa fever is the commonest cause of pericarditis in Sierra Leone. Blood tests are as shown in this case, with a normal clotting screen and platelet count, and if the AST is very high as in this case, the mortality is around 55%. Ribavirin will reduce this mortality to around 5%.

The second week is crucial in this illness, with the patient either surviving with an average total duration of illness of 15 days, or going on to die from shock, and encephalitis manifested by grand mal fits after 12 days of illness. In the survivors, alopecia and sensorineural deafness are common.

During the second week, there is lower abdominal pain, vomiting, swelling, hypotension and bleeding. The bleeding tendency is relatively slight and is not enough to account for the shock. For example, a small amount of bleeding may occur from the gums. Petechiae or haemorrhagic rashes are not seen. Chest X-rays can show basal shadows or pleural effusions, ECG changes can occur and as in this case, the creatine kinase can be elevated.

The diagnosis is made either by isolation of the virus in specialist centres or demonstrating a rise in titre of antibodies to Lassa fever virus and the illness is very unlikely if IgM antibodies are not detected by 2 weeks after the onset of the illness. Extreme caution is required in handling blood from these patients and special techniques are needed for laboratory safety. Standard ward isolation procedures have controlled epidemics in Africa and there have not been any cases of secondary transmission of Lassa fever so far in the United Kingdom.

Various other haemorrhagic fevers can occur in Africa, Europe, South America, South East Asia and Siberia. They are transmitted by arthropods (arboviruses) or rodents (roboviruses).

Table 1 shows the most common arboviral haemorrhagic fevers.

Table 1: Arboviral fevers and their vectors

Russian spring–summer encephalitis	tick
Crimean-Congo haemorrhagic fever	tick
Dengue	mosquito
Chikungunya	mosquito
Yellow fever	mosquito

Zoonotic arboviruses are Hantaan (a bunyavirus), Junin and Machupo viruses from South America, Lassa fever and probably Ebola virus (Filovirus). The exact mode of transmission of Ebola is still unknown but it is presumed to be a robovirus.

Most haemorrhagic fever viruses produce fever, petechiae or

purpura, bleeding from the GI tract or vagina, shock, neutropenia, thrombocytopenia and proteinuria. The patient oftens dies from acute encephalopathy. Hantaan virus produces haemorrhagic fever with a renal syndrome (HFRS) and the disease is particularly severe in Korea with a mortality of around 10%. A Hantaan-related virus has been isolated from the domestic rat in the United States and although Hantaan virus itself is not a clinical problem in the USA, 6% of longshore men in Baltimore have neutralizing antibodies to the virus. There is currently much interest in a new Hantaan-like virus ('sin nombre') in the USA that causes rapidly fatal ARDS.

Junin haemorrhagic fever has a mortality of 10–15% in untreated cases and it is a particular problem in the rich agricultural regions of Argentina, affecting workers in cereal fields. It produces a temporary impairment of cell mediated immune responses and causes death by secondary infections.

Machupo virus is found in Bolivia, but no large epidemics have been seen since a major rodent control effort, except for some isolated ranches.

Ebola virus causes the typical syndrome of fever, shock and death. It starts with prostration followed by diarrhoea and vomiting. Convalescent plasma from survivors has been used in treatment, which is otherwise supportive. Outbreaks have been seen in Sudan and Zaire and in fact the Ebola river is in Zaire. The fatality rate can be up to 80%, and hospital staff run high risks in epidemics. Unfortunately, despite extensive efforts the reservoir for this virus is still unknown, so an elimination campaign is not possible.

The Ebola virus attracts a considerable amount of publicity in the United Kingdom, and when outbreaks occur in Africa the index of suspicion in returning travellers is very high. Therefore, reading the guidelines issued by the Department of Health or the Welsh Office is essential for all those concerned with managing infectious diseases, and expert help should be sought as soon as the diagnosis is suspected.

Further reading

McCormick, J. B., Webb, P. A., Krebs, J. W. et al. (1987) A prospective study of the epidemiology and ecology of Lassa fever. J. Infect. Dis., **155**, 437.

Case 15   Sneezing, headache and a convulsion

A 14-year-old girl went on a summer camping trip to the New Forest with her parents and 10-year-old brother. She developed a sore throat, runny nose and sneezing which the parents attributed to her seasonal hay fever. Over the next week, her symptoms fluctuated and treatment with antihistamines and paracetamol for fever were continued. She then began to complain of a severe throbbing headache and night sweats and 12 days after the onset of symptoms she developed a convulsion and was rushed to a nearby hospital. On admission, her temperature was 38.8°C, heart rate 90/min, blood pressure 130/70 mmHg and respiratory rate 24/min. She was irritable and examination revealed tenderness to percussion over the forehead. There was blurring of the right optic disk and an emergency CT scan was requested.

Questions

1. What is the potentially fatal diagnosis?
2. What pathogens are expected?
3. What is the treatment of this condition?

Answers

1. The immediate consideration is of a frontal lobe brain abscess arising from contiguous frontal sinusitis. The symptoms of allergic rhinitis can be identical to infected sinusitis and to confound matters, the former can give rise to the latter. Disruption of normal ciliary clearance mechanisms and obstruction of sinus ostia by mucus from allergic conditions or viral upper respiratory tract infection allows growth of respiratory flora in the affected sinus with the occurrence of a bacterial sinusitis. Spread from the sinus to contiguous brain areas occurs through local lymphatics and penetrating (emissary) veins. The CT scan did in fact show an enhancing lesion in the right frontal lobe. This case illustrates the speed with which such abscesses can develop from underlying sinusitis.
2. The organisms to be expected in this brain abscess are those found in the acutely infected frontal sinus. The sinus infection is usually polymicrobial with anaerobic and microaerophilic

streptococci, *Bacteroides sp.* and *Fusobacterium sp.* It is vitally important that empirical choices of antimicrobials for a brain abscess take into consideration the expected pathogens in a given patient. Chronic middle ear disease, for example, raises the possibility of *Proteus* sp., other *enterobacteriaceae* and *Pseudomonas sp.* in addition.

3. The treatment of brain abscess is with appropriate antimicrobials, preferably after surgical aspiration or excision of the lesion. Antimicrobials chosen must cover all expected pathogens in a given case and achieve high enough levels in the abscess cavity. Whether or not surgery is employed depends on the following:

   (i) The likely underlying conditions and range of expected pathogens.

   (ii) The size of the lesion; abscesses smaller than 4 cm are more likely to respond to antimicrobials alone.

   (iii) Deterioration of clinical status or enlargement of an abscess on sequential CT studies.

Many authorities believe that surgical aspiration should always be considered, since it reduces mass effect and provides material for laboratory stains, culture and sensitivity testing of isolates. This patient was treated with high dose parenteral cefotaxime and metronidazole empirically. *Benzylpenicillin* was also given when Gram stain of subsequently aspirated pus from the abscess showed Gram positive cocci in chains. Culture revealed Group A beta-haemolytic streptococci *(S. pyogenes)* and *Peptostreptococcus* sp.

Further reading

Szuwart, U. and Bennefeld, H. (1990) Bacteriological analysis of pyogenic infections of the brain. *Neurosurg. Rev.*, **13**, 113.

Case 16 A cervical mass lesion with cord compression in a diabetic

A 45-year-old diabetic man previously in good health presented to the general medical outpatients clinic with neck pain.

He had been well until 4 weeks previously when he apparently 'jolted' his neck when stopping his car suddenly. He then developed pain in the cervical region which radiated to the left shoulder. Plain neck radiographs requested by his general practitioner revealed no evidence of fracture or displacement. Routine blood tests performed by the GP showed a normal haemoglobin and white cell count, but an ESR of 50 mm/h. A serum biochemical profile was normal and he did not have a fever. In the clinic he denied any further symptoms but complained that the neck pain had worsened. Examination revealed spasm of the muscles in the neck and limitation of movement in all directions. There was local tenderness over the C4 and C5 spinous processes, but the remainder of the CNS examination was normal. Examination of heart, chest and abdomen revealed no abnormality.

An MRI of the cervical region was obtained as an emergency which revealed an abnormal segment in the posterior part of the C4 vertebral body, and an abnormal segment in the posterior part of the C4/5 intervertebral disc. The disc base was narrowed and there was an area of diminished attenuation bulging into the spinal canal causing cord compression anteriorly over the area of the C4 and C5 vertebrae.

Questions

1. What is the likely infective diagnosis?
2. You are asked to advise – what do you recommend?

Answers

1. Anterior cervical epidural abscess possibly complicating vertebral osteomyelitis.
2. Immediate surgery to drain the abscess and to evacuate infection from bone.

Comment

An epidural abscess should be considered in any case where localized back pain occurs with radiation. Local tenderness and rigidity of the neck are very characteristic and epidural abscesses occur in the cervical region in around 15% of cases. The epidural abscess usually occupies four or five vertebral segments or may extend even further. This is because in the spinal canal the dura mater is separated from the vertebrae by fat filled epidural space and there is therefore no resistance to the longitudinal spread of infection. Within the narrow space of the spinal canal, enlargement of the abscess can produce cord necrosis, both by compression and possibly by sudden vascular thrombosis. An epidural abscess can be present without a fever or leucocytosis as in this case, but the raised ESR should not be seen following uncomplicated trauma. It was the presence of radicular pain that made this patient an emergency and the diagnostic procedure of choice for an epidural abscess is MRI as it allows visualization of the vertebrae also, and the vertebrae are found to be involved in 90% of cases. Bacterial infection very often affects the posterior parts of vertebral bodies, and may also affect the avascular intervertebral discs. Tumours very rarely cross the disc, as a good blood supply is necessary for their spread.

Because of the danger of spinal cord necrosis, surgical drainage is usually required but antibiotics should be given prior to surgery. *Staphyloccocus aureus* causes 70% of cases, with aerobic and anaerobic streptococci causing a further 8% of cases.

A small number of patients have been treated using CT guided aspiration instead of laminectomy but if antibiotic therapy alone is used the patient requires intensive monitoring and repeated MRI scans. In the presence of worsening pain and fever or the appearance of a neurological deficit urgent surgery should be performed.

The outcome is excellent if therapy begins when radicular symptoms are present without spinal cord injury. In a case such as this where osteomyelitis was also present, antibiotic therapy should be continued for another 8 weeks.

Further reading

LASTER, B. R. and HARTER, D. H. (1987) Cervical epidural abscess. *Neurology*, **37**, 1747.

Case 17 A pregnant paediatric nurse with a skin rash

A 24-year-old nurse was 17 weeks pregnant and working on the paediatric oncology unit. She had been assigned to nurse an immunocompetent child with chickenpox, as she had herself suffered from confirmed chickenpox as a child. Ten days after the child was discharged she developed a diffuse rash and fever, and she remained at home. Three days after the appearance of the rash she developed a non-productive cough, pleuritic chest pain and shortness of breath. Her general practitioner was called, and she was admitted to hospital. There was no significant past medical history except the usual childhood illnesses and she had no children. Her husband was well and worked as a painter and decorator and there were no household pets.

On examination her respiratory rate was 30/min, temperature 39°C, blood pressure 110/70, pulse 120/min. A vesicular and pustular rash was seen on her trunk. Examination of the chest showed fine inspiratory crackles bilaterally. Examination of heart, abdomen and central nervous system were normal. Urinalysis was normal.

Blood results were Hb 13.1 g/dl, WBC 14.5×10^9/l (65% neutrophils), sodium 140 mmol/l, potassium 3.6 mmol/l, urea 3.0 mmol/l, creatinine 76 μmol/l. The AST was raised at 140 IU/l, and the alkaline phosphatase was raised at 123 IU/l but the other liver function tests were normal. Blood gases on air were; pO_2 64 mmHg, pCO_2 30 mmHg, pH 7.47. A chest X-ray showed bilateral basal alveolar and interstitial shadows and she was given oxygen.

Questions

1. What is the diagnosis?
2. What treatment should be given?

Answers

1. Varicella pneumonitis
2. Intravenous acyclovir.

Comment

The varicella zoster virus is a member of the herpesvirus family, and transmission is most likely by inhalation. There may be replication at an unidentified site in the body, followed by a viraemia leading to scattered skin lesions. Vesicles occur initially, but they become cloudy with the arrival of neutrophils, and on bursting they release the infectious virus. Some blood vessels can be affected directly, leading to necrosis and haemorrhage in the skin. Chickenpox will affect 90% of exposed non-immune individuals and half of all cases are in children between the age of 5 and 9 years. The incubation period is usually around 2 weeks, but ranges from 10 days to 3 weeks. The duration of infectivity (which is a common query in the control of hospital infection) is from 2 days prior to the first appearance of the rash, for the next 5 days of vesicle formation, and until all the lesions are crusted over. There is occasionally a prodromal illness, but most often there is not. Although chickenpox is a harmless illness in the normal child, children with leukaemia or other causes of immunosuppression such as steroid treatment can develop very many lesions (some with a haemorrhagic base) and healing takes around three times longer than normal. Around 15% of patients with leukaemia who contract chickenpox will die.

The complications of varicella include an acute cerebellar ataxia most commonly occurring around 3 weeks after the start of the rash. It is benign and requires no treatment. Other complications include aseptic meningitis, encephalitis, transverse myelitis, Reye's syndrome and hepatitis. The AST is often raised, as in this case, and is of no significance.

The most severe complication of infection is varicella pneumonitis and this can occur in around 20% of adults with chickenpox. Between 3 and 5 days after the start of illness, there is an increased respiratory rate, cough, shortness of breath, fever and very often chest pain and haemoptysis. Chest X-rays will show nodular infiltrates and pneumonitis. Although the X-ray appearance most commonly improves with improvement in the rash, occasionally patients can be extremely ill for many weeks. The pneumonitis can prove fatal despite acyclovir and ventilation and there is a place for extracorporeal membrane oxygenation (ECMO) which may be life saving. Patients with pneumonitis of this severity should be investigated subsequently for immune deficiencies such as immunoglobulin subclass deficiencies.

In pregnancy, varicella pneumonia can be very serious and has been reported to have a mortality of 44% in some studies. This may be related to the immunosuppression that occurs in pregnancy and of course the splinting of the chest in late pregnancy may also contribute to hypoxia. Taking studies as a whole, without antiviral therapy mortality is around 36%, but since the discovery of acyclovir the prognosis has improved markedly with a reported fatality of 13%. The doses that have been used are around 500 mg tds intravenously and no side-effects have been noted.

The frequency of intra-uterine infection with varicella appears to increase with the duration of pregnancy but the risk of con-genital defects from varicella seems to occur in the first trimester. Overall, congenital problems are extremely rare. On acyclovir treatment, fetal loss was related to the death of the mother, and if the mother survived the fetus was born normally.

There is a great risk to the child if the mother is infected with chickenpox from the period of 2 days prior to delivery to 5 days after delivery. This is because the mother has not been able to synthesize protective antibody and passively immunize the child. The mortality for the child in this situation is around 30% and this is an indication to give the mother acyclovir. If the mother contracts chickenpox 7 days prior to, or up to a month after delivery, the baby should be given varicella-zoster immune globulin (VZIG) as prophylaxis. There is no evidence that VZIG is useful in actual disease. VZIG should also be given to immunosuppressed patients considered at risk of developing chickenpox, including those who have been taking high dose steroids for more than 1 week in the previous 3 months.

Only 5% of women between the ages of 15 and 40 lack IgG antibodies to varicella zoster virus, because the disease is so common in childhood and so contagious. This patient represents a re-infection with chickenpox which has been shown to occur occasionally and therefore the possibility of chickenpox pneumonitis should not be ruled out even with definite history of previous exposure. For routine purposes, patients with a definite previous history of chickenpox should not be considered at risk even if immunosuppressed, but if the patient is under 15, immunosuppressed and has an unknown history of chickenpox then VZIG should be given after significant contact with chickenpox. A varicella vaccine is under development which is available on a named-patient basis from SmithKline Beecham, or Merieux.

Further reading

GERSHON, A. A. (1992) Varicella vaccine: still at the crossroads. *Pediatrics*, **90**, 144–148.

Case 18   Intensive care and infection

A 60-year-old male was admitted to the Cardiac Intensive Care Unit following aortic valve replacement and ventilated. He developed post-operative pneumonia diagnosed by chest X-ray changes, pyrexia and overall clinical deterioration, and was treated empirically with cefotaxime and metronidazole. One week later, he became febrile again and blood cultures grew a coagulase-negative staphylococcus in samples from a central venous line and from a peripheral vein. Teicoplanin was added to the antibiotic regimen and all lines were changed. Four days later the patient again developed a fever. Blood cultures were drawn and therapy was changed to ciprofloxacin and teicoplanin. The most recent blood cultures were positive after 24 h and the Gram-stain showed small, coccoid Gram-negative rods. A review of all microbiology data showed:

   (i) An endotracheal aspirate taken early in his illness had grown a proteus species sensitive to cefotaxime.
  (ii) Coagulase-negative staphylococci grown from blood cultures – methicillin resistant, teicoplanin and vancomycin sensitive.
 (iii) Culture of a recent endotracheal sample had a moderate growth of an oxidase-negative Gram-negative coccobacillus growing well on blood agar. The organism showed good growth on MacConkey agar and produced a lavender tint.
  (iv) The prevailing gram-negative bacteria on the Intensive Care Unit were *Enterobacter sp.* and a recent increase in multi-resistant *Acinetobacter sp.*, following the admission of a colonized patient.

Questions

1. What is the likely organism now in the blood?
2. What is the drug of choice?

3. What factors contribute to the patient becoming colonized with this organism prior to the development of bacteraemia?

Answers

1. The features described for the organism are typical of *Acinetobacter* sp. – the Gram-stain showing cocco-bacilli (diplococcal forms may occur) and oxidase negativity. The good growth on blood agar and on MacConkey agar with a lavender or blue tint of the colonies are also characteristic. *Acinetobacter* can be divided into at least 12 groups known as genospecies based on DNA homology studies. *Acinetobacter baumanii* (genospecies 2) is the species most commonly found in clinical samples and can be identified by the API system.

2. The organism can be multi-resistant but tends to maintain sensitivity to imipenem, which is the drug of choice. Some authorities recommend combination therapy with a beta-lactam such as imipenem or ceftazidime and an aminoglycoside for potential synergy.

3. This case illustrates many of the features which predispose a patient to *Acinetobacter* colonization and subsequent invasion. These include the major surgery, intensive care environment, treatment with multiple antimicrobials, mechanical ventilation and proximity to patients harbouring the organism. The organism grows well in the moist environment of ventilator tubing and sinks but outbreaks have also been traced to dry formites such as pillows and mattresses. The use of broad-spectrum antimicrobials exerts a positive selection pressure once multiple resistance has developed. Most infections are hospital-acquired and include bacteraemia, pneumonia, endocarditis, meningitis and urinary tract infections. Cutaneous lesions can be readily colonized and occasionally, even normal skin. In the present case there appears to have been an antecedent pneumonia and the bacteraemia may have arisen from this or through a colonized intravascular catheter. In choosing empirical treatment for a patient on the ICU with, say, suspected Gram-negative sepsis, consider:

   (i) The potential sources of infection, e.g. vascular lines.
   (ii) The potential anatomical locations of the infection, e.g. pneumonia.

(iii) The antimicrobial and microbiologic history of the patient.
(iv) The surrounding flora: what are the prevailing organisms on the unit? Which organisms are colonizing nearby patients?

Further reading

BERGOGNE-BEREZIN, E. and JOLY-GUILLOU, M. L. (1986) Comparative activity of imipenem, ceftazidime and cefotaxime against *Acinetobacter calcoaceticus. J. Antimicrob. Chemother.*, **18** (Suppl E), 35.

Case 19   A young student from Mozambique with haematuria

A 20-year-old male student who was a native of Mozambique presented to the outpatient department with a 6-month history of dysuria and haematuria. There was a history of suprapubic pain but no history of fever, chills, nausea or vomiting. Urethral swabs for gonorrhoea and chlamydia were negative as was culture of the urine for significant bacteriuria. On examination, the vital signs were normal; there was no lymphadenopathy and the abdomen was normal apart from some minimal suprapubic tenderness. There were venereal warts on the glans penis. Laboratory investigation showed: haemoglobin 16.7 g/dl, WBC 7.0×10^9/l with 73% polymorphs, 21% lymphs, 2% monocytes, 3% eosinophils, 1% basophils. Urinalysis showed: protein +, blood +++, 21–40 white cells, and large numbers of red cells/hpf. Further microscopy of the urine after concentration showed identifiable structures.

Questions

1. What is the likely diagnosis?
2. What is the treatment of choice?

Answers

1. The likely diagnosis is chronic schistosomiasis of the urinary

tract, based both on the clinical features and epidemiology of the disease, and this was in fact confirmed by the urine microscopy showing eggs of *S. haematobium*. This organism produces a granulomatous inflammation of the urinary tract. The main clinical features of chronic disease are haematuria, dysuria and frequency with associated laboratory evidence of haematuria and proteinuria. Thickening of the bladder wall and obstructive uropathy are frequent findings and this patient had a right hydro-ureter and hydronephrosis on intra-venous pyelography. Further complications of chronic disease are pyelonephritis and carcinoma of the urinary bladder.

2. The drug of choice for all species of schistosoma is praziquantel. It is administered as two oral doses for the treatment of *S. haematobium*. Follow-up examination of the urine should be performed several weeks after therapy to ensure that there are no viable eggs. Praziquantel may reverse very early pathological lesions but not established fibrosis or the associated obstructive processes.

Comment

Schistosomiasis caused by *S. haematobium, S. mansoni, S. japonicum, S. mekongi* and *S. intercalatum* occurs throughout Africa, Asia and South America, wherever the species specific snail intermediate hosts are found. Man is the principal definitive host and clinical features whether of acute or chronic disease, reflect the stages of development of these parasites in the host, producing schistosome dermatitis, Katayama fever or chronic obstructive syndromes. Diagnosis requires enquiry about travel and suggestive clinical features and, appropriate specimens for laboratory detection of eggs, e.g. faeces, urine or rectal biopsy. For *S. haematobium,* urine is best collected between 12 noon and 2 p.m. Serological tests are available but must be interpreted with care particularly in persons from an endemic area.

Further reading

KING, C. H. and MAHMOUD, A. A. F. (1989) Drugs five years later: praziquantel. *Ann. Int. Med.*, **110**, 290.

Case 20   A male homosexual with a cerebellar lesion

A 39-year-old homosexual electrician had been diagnosed 3 months earlier has having antibodies to HIV-1. At that time he was noted to have necrotizing gingivitis and seborrhoeic dermatitis, and he complained of a headache. A contrast enhanced CT scan of the head was normal and a lumbar puncture revealed cryptococci. He was treated with intravenous amphotericin and flucytosine, and subsequently with oral fluconazole. His CD4 count was known to be 40/mm^3 and he had a normochromic normocytic anaemia. He was prescribed Septrin for prophylaxis against *Pneumocystis carinii* as well as fluconazole for prophylaxis against cryptococcosis. One week before admission he had difficulty in walking and clumsiness of the left hand.

Physical examination revealed an apyrexial thin man with gingivitis but no candidiasis. The chest and abdomen were clear. There was nystagmus on leftward gaze and poor finger-nose coordination and poor heel-shin manoeuvre on the left. There were no pyramidal signs or sensory disturbances. He had no fever and the conscious level was normal.

Blood results were: HB 10.0 g/dl, WBC 4.4×10^9/l platelets 113×10^9/l, urea and electrolytes normal. The ESR was normal. Serological tests for toxoplasma and VDRL/TPHA were negative. An MRI scan of the brain showed a lesion in the left middle cerebellar peduncle with no mass effect and no enhancement after gadolinium. The lesion was reported to resemble an area of demyelination.

Questions

1. What is the probable diagnosis?
2. What further tests would you perform on the CSF?

Answers

1. Progressive multifocal leukencephalopathy
2. Culture for viruses such as CMV, VZV, HSV-1, HSV-2, toxoplasma antibodies and toxoplasma PCR, VDRL/TPHA and PCR for JC virus.

Comment

Progressive multifocal leukencephalopathy (PML) is the result of infection of oligodendrocytes with a papovavirus known as JC. This results in demyelinization in discrete areas of the brain accompanied by enlarged astrocytes and enlargement of oligodendroglial nuclei and these nuclei are seen to contain papovavirus-like particles on electron microscopy. The JC virus does not infect neurones directly. By the age of 10 years, 50% of normal individuals have antibodies to JC virus and PML is the consequence of reactivation in those individuals who become immunosuppressed. The virus is spread in the normal population by the respiratory route.

PML occurs in around 4% of patients with AIDS and clinically the diagnosis is suspected where a focal neurological syndrome is accompanied by imaging of the brain which shows disease in the white matter without mass affect. Often the patient presents with a hemiparesis and in 10% of cases ataxia results from involvement of the cerebellum. As the disease advances, extrapyramidal symptoms may occur. Patients may also present with homonymous hemianopia due to lesions of the optic radiation, and around 6% of patients have cortical blindness as the presenting feature of PML. There may be rapidly developing personality and behavioural changes along with memory impairment. Only 10% of patients show a sensory deficit.

Although the diagnosis of PML is definitively made by brain biopsy, supporting evidence can be gleaned from CT scanning that shows hypodense lesions in areas of white matter. These are non-enhancing and do not have a mass effect. On MRI, T2 weighted images may show hyperintense lesions and again there is no enhancement with contrast in 95% of cases. The diagnosis of PML should not be dismissed if the cortical regions are not affected, as 7% of patients have disease restricted to the posterior fossa (as in this case).

Although the AIDS dementia complex can be accompanied by similar radiographic appearances, the clinical course is very different. Not only is PML much more rapidly progressive but it also gives rise to *focal* neurological signs. Cytomegalovirus can also cause demyelinating lesions but these are typically located in the white matter surrounding the ventricles. In this case, the speed of progression can be judged from the previous normal CT scan a few months earlier, and the outlook for the patient is very poor, with death expected in around 4 months. However, around 8% of patients with biopsy proven PML can improve spontaneously and this makes assessment of proposed treatments, such as cytarabine, very difficult. The cerebrospinal fluid protein may be elevated, and in 30% of cases will be positive for the JC virus by PCR. However, the specificity of this result is currently unknown. Brain biopsy demonstrating demyelinization and abnormal nuclei in astrocytes is still the only diagnostic method.

The patient deteriorated quickly and died. Post-mortem examination revealed extensive PML of the cerebellum and also small regions of demyelinization scattered over the cerebral grey matter that were not seen on MRI.

Further reading

BERGER, J. R., KASZOVITZ, B., POST, M. J. *et al.* (1987) Progressive multifocal leukoencephalopathy associated with human immunodeficiency virus infection. A review of the literature with a report of sixteen cases. *Ann. Intern. Med.*, **107**, 78–87.

Case 21 Late neonatal fever

A 5-week-old female child was admitted to hospital with poor feeding, pyrexia and lethargy. This was the 28-year-old mother's first pregnancy, and normal delivery followed membrane rupture by 2 h. An ante-natal screen in the last trimester for Group B streptococcal carriage was positive and the mother was treated with amoxycillin for 2 weeks prior to delivery. On admission, blood cultures and a sample of CSF were obtained from the child. The CSF was normal biochemically and was sterile after 3 days incubation. Blood cultures were positive after 24 h for a Gram-positive coccus in chains.

Questions

1. What is the likely diagnosis?
2. What other tests are available for the laboratory diagnosis of Group B streptococcal sepsis?

3. What is your approach to Group B streptococcal carriage in pregnancy?

Answers

1. The immediate diagnosis to be considered is late-onset Group B streptococcal sepsis with bacteraemia. Although most cases of late onset disease also involve the meninges, this case illustrates the exception. It also shows that anti-microbial prophylaxis for the mother may only delay the onset of Group B sepsis in the child. Group B streptococci (GBS) can be serotyped into types 1a, 1b, II and III. The antepartum isolate from the mother was unavailable, but she was found to be an anal carrier of type III and her child was also infected with type III.
2. Latex agglutination tests are available for detection of GBS antigen in serum, CSF and urine. These tests must follow the specific manufacturer's recommendations for optimal sensitivity and specificity. Urine may be concentrated to increase sensitivity, which approaches 75% overall.
3. This issue is still being debated because of the frequency and serious sequelae of Group B infection in neonates. The consensus is that prophylaxis should only be employed for high risk deliveries, i.e. women who are GBS carriers *and* who have one or more risk factors for development of GBS disease in the new-born (premature labour, prolonged rupture of membranes, or peripartum fever). If there are risk factors but the maternal Group B status is unknown, there may be a case for prophylaxis if time precludes culture or if rapid tests for detection of carriage have low sensitivities. Intrapartum prophylaxis appears to be the most cost-effective, since the antimicrobial employed (e.g. ampicillin) achieves high levels in the neonate as well as the mother.

Further reading

PASS, M. A., GRAY, B. M., KHARE, S. *et al.* (1979) Prospective studies of group B streptococcal infections in infants. *J. Pediatr.*, **95**, 437–443.

Case 22   A man with joint pains and weight loss

A 48-year-old Italian waiter was seen in the outpatient clinic complaining of 4 months of weight loss, abdominal pain and diarrhoea. The diarrhoea was described as watery and offensive, and he was passing up to six loose stools a day with no blood. The abdominal pain was epigastric and more severe after meals.

Ten years previously had been seen by the rheumatologists for joint pains that were fleeting in nature, lasting 1–4 days in a given area. The areas most affected were the ankles, knees, shoulders and wrists. There was no joint deformity and he was still occasionally using non-steroidal anti-inflammatory agents. He believed that he had been suffering from 'fevers' for the past year. He was of Italian descent but born in the UK

On examination he appeared to have suffered loss of weight, was hypotensive (BP 100/60), and there was a low grade fever at 37.8°C. Pulse was 80/min; the abdomen was slightly distended and tender on palpation. There was no organomegaly but small axillary and inguinal lymph nodes were readily detectable.

Investigation showed Hb 9.1 g/dl, MCV 65 fl, WBC $9.2 \times 10^9/l$, platelets $593 \times 10^9/l$, ESR 52 mm/h, serum iron 9 (50–150), sodium 137 mmol/l, potassium 4.9 mmol/l. Urea, creatinine, calcium, and phosphate were normal, and liver function tests were normal apart from a slightly raised alkaline phosphate. The albumin was 30 g/l, thyroid function was normal, and tests for rheumatoid factor, antinuclear factor and VDRL were negative. Microscopy of stool for parasites and cultures of blood and urine were all negative. An HIV test was negative.

A chest X-ray was normal and an upper gastrointestinal barium study showed thickened duodenal folds. Proctoscopy and rectal biopsy were normal. A collection of stool showed 23 g of fat/24 h (normal < 5.5/24 h) and a d-xylose absorption test showed 2.5 g excreted for 5 h after a 25 g oral dose (normal > 4.2 g).

Questions

1. What is the organism responsible for this illness?
2. What is the treatment?
3. What is the diagnostic procedure?

Answers

1. *Tropheryma whippelii.*
2. Antibiotic therapy.
3. Diagnosis would be made by small bowel biopsy and PAS staining.

Comment

In 1907, G. H. Whipple described a 36-year-old patient with loss of weight and strength, stools consisting of fat, indefinite abdominal signs and 'peculiar multiple arthritis'. Using silver stains, Whipple described vacuoles containing 'rod shaped organisms' rarely exceeding 2 microns in length but fairly numerous. By electron microscopy, we now know that microorganisms are present in macrophages in Whipple's disease and that these microorganisms disappear following treatment with antibiotics such as penicillin and tetracycline. Although the bowel is most affected, these bacteria have been seen in the nervous system, heart, synovial tissue, lymph nodes, lung and liver. It seems that a single bacterial strain is responsible for all cases, and in 1991 and 1992 work on the sequences of the 16S ribosomal RNA genes allowed the classification of the organism as a Gram-positive actinomycete, not closely related to any of the known species. The positive staining with PAS is consistent with many actinomyces. In 1992, the name *Tropheryma whippelii* was suggested as a tribute to Whipple and the recognition that malabsorption is a major symptom (trope is Greek for nourishment).

Gastrointestinal manifestations of Whipple's disease include diarrhoea in 75% of cases, usually watery and associated with steatorrhoea. There is non-specific abdominal pain and bloating. Eight-two per cent of patients have arthritis for a mean of 9 years before presentation and weight loss occurs in 89% of patients for a mean of 8 months before presentation. Around half the patients have had fever for more than 4 years. Peripheral joints are the most often involved and the disease can resemble palindromic rheumatism but with a negative rheumatoid factor and lack of metacarpophalangeal joint involvement. The skin can be dark as in pellagra or carcinoid, and lung involvement can lead to a chronic cough. Heart involvement can lead to heart failure pericarditis.

Ten per cent of patients with Whipple's disease have neurological involvement, and this can present with supranuclear ophthalmopathy, nystagmus, bruxism and myoclonic ocular and facial jerks. It can cause a parkinsonian syndrome and the MRI will show white matter changes that are enchanced by gadolinium. Involvement of the CNS means that antibiotics used for treatment should be able to penetrate the blood–brain barrier. Endoscopy can show white plaques and erosions in the duodenum and this is the commonest cause of iron deficiency anaemia, although this patient had been taking non-steroidals also.

Physical examination may reveal hyperpigmentation, hypotension and in hypoalbuminaemia, ascites and peripheral oedema. Lymphadenopathy is present in 50% of cases, usually firm and non-tender. Endocardial infiltration by the bacteria can cause valvular stenosis or incompetence, and a periumbilical mass may be felt due to enlarged mesenteric lymph nodes. Central nervous system examination may show dementia, confusion, cranial nerve abnormalities, ataxia or peripheral neuropathy. The most common laboratory abnormalities are steatorrhoea, hypoalbuminaemia, iron deficiency anaemia and a raised ESR. The differential diagnosis in this case would involve the causes of 'enteropathic arthritis' (see Table 1).

Table 1: The differential diagnosis of enteropathic arthritis

1.	Inflammatory bowel disease (IBD)
2.	Reiter's syndrome
3.	Familial Mediterranean fever
4.	Polyarteritis nodosa
5.	Behcet's syndrome

The arthritis of IBD predominantly involves the lower extremities, especially the knees and ankles. It is often migratory and rarely destructive. In this case, arthralgia preceded the onset of gastrointestinal symptoms by several years, and proctoscopy did not identify colitis. Reiter's syndrome can follow enteric infections with *shigella, salmonella, campylobacter* and *yersinia*. Reiter's usually involves lower extremity joints but symptoms resolve within weeks or months in 90% of cases. Again it is unusual for arthritis to precede the diarrhoea. Also, this patient had no conjunctivitis, urethritis or mucocutaneous lesions. Fever, arthralgia and abdominal pain in an Italian patient should suggest familial Mediterranean fever, which produces attacks of fever, abdominal, chest and joint pain, and painful skin nodules on the leg. These attacks last 24–48 h. In this case, the diarrhoea was prominent and there were no attacks of acute abdominal or chest pain. Polyarteritis nodosa (PAN) is unlikely due to the lack of renal involvement or hypertension, and also the 5-year survival of PAN is only 10%.

Duodenal biopsy would show that the villi were clubbed in appearance with flattening and vacuolization of absorptive cells. There would be numerous fat droplets throughout the lamina propria and there would be intense PAS staining.

The HIV test in this case was negative; it would be important to think of HIV infection complicated by *Mycobacterium avium intracellulare* infection in the scenario presented. *M. avium* also stains with PAS, but will also be AFB positive whereas AFB stains in Whipple's disease are negative.

Further reading

RELMAN, D. A., SCHMIDT, T. M., MACDERMOTT, R. P. *et al.* (1992) Identification of the uncultured bacillus of Whipple's disease. *N. Engl. J. Med.*, **327**, 293–296.

Case 23   Hodgkin's disease with headache and fever

A 65-year-old male with a history of Hodgkin's disease in remission presented with acute severe generalized headache. He gave a history of associated double vision and was pyrexial to 38.5°C on admission. A lumbar puncture and blood cultures were performed and he was commenced on cefotaxime 2 g tds. The lumbar puncture showed: WBC $20\,000 \times 10^9/l$ (polymorphs 97%), Gram-stain – Gram positive rods (skinny as opposed to fatter *Bacillus sp.*, for example)

Questions

1. What is the likely diagnosis?
2. How should therapy be altered?

3. What are the expected features of the organism if and when grown?

Answers

1. The likely diagnosis is meningitis with or without bacteraemia from *Listeria monocytogenes*. Although some patients who develop non-perinatal listeriosis have no apparent immunocompromising conditions, most are in fact immunocompromised from underlying disease or therapy.
2. The cephalosporins should not be used for the treatment of listeriosis. Ampicillin plus gentamicin is still a favoured combination because of possible synergy and can be added to the cefotaxime pending confirmation of the diagnosis by culture of the CSF. Treatment should be for 2–4 weeks.
3. Amongst the species of *Listeria*, virtually all human disease is caused by *L. monocytogenes*. This organism is a thin grampositive rod which can be easily confused with 'diphtheroids' (skin corynebacteria) and vice versa. On blood agar, the organism shows beta-haemolysis. Organisms grown in broth cultures at 20–25°C show 'tumbling' motility (like a pencil being twirled about its mid-point). Final biochemical identification can be done using an API gram-positive panel.

Comment

It is always important to extract as much information as possible from initial laboratory data as this may have a greater impact on patient management and clinical outcome than the final laboratory result. In this regard, priority smears, such as those on sterile body fluids, should be reviewed by clinicians and laboratory staff in immediate joint consultation. Skill in Gram-stained smear interpretation (to varying degrees) should be the goal of all post-graduate clinical trainees.

Further reading

GELLIN, B. G. and BROOME, C. V. (1989) Listeriosis. *JAMA*, **262**, 1313.

Case 24 A male homosexual with a dilated heart

A 40-year-old homosexual man was admitted to hospital complaining of shortness of breath, muscles pains and progressive weakness.

He had been well until 2 years earlier when he developed *Pnemocystis carinii* pneumonia and was found to be HIV positive. That infection was treated with co-trimoxazole and he was thereafter maintained on prophylactic aerosolized pentamidine as he had developed a rash on taking Septrin. He had been taking Zidovudine (AZT) for the previous 10 months and was also taking acyclovir for recurrent perianal herpes simplex and fluconazole for oral candidiasis. He had lost some weight in the month prior to admission and he did not complain of headache.

On examination the temperature was 40°C, pulse 130/min and BP 110/60. The jugular venous pressure was raised, and on auscultation a summation gallop was found. There were basal crackles bilaterally and the liver edge could be felt 4 cm below the costal margin, but the spleen could not be palpated. Neurological examination was normal apart from general muscle weakness. Examination of the ocular fundi was normal.

Blood results were Hb 10.0 g/dl, WBC 2.1 ×10^9/l, MCV 92 fl, platelets 84 × 10^9/l, ESR 57 mm/h, clotting screen normal, sodium 135 mmol/l, potassium 4.0 mmol/l, urea 11.0 mmol/l, creatinine 120 μmol/l, albumin 21 g/l, AST 180 IU/l (10–40), creatine kinase 1100 IU/l (<250), CKMB isoenzyme normal. Culture of blood, urine and stool gave negative results for viruses, bacteria and mycobacteria. IgG antibody to toxoplasma was present and the IgM antibody was negative. Cryptococcal antigen was negative in the serum.

Chest X-ray showed cardiomegaly with upper lobe venous diversion and an ECG showed sinus tachycardia. An X-ray film of the abdomen showed hepatosplenomegaly and CT scan of the brain was normal. The CSF was clear with no growth of cryptococcus, herpesviruses or bacteria including *Listeria*.

Echocardiography showed dilatation of all cardiac chambers and hypokinesis of the interventricular septum. Bronchoalveolar lavage showed no evidence of pneumocystis or cryptococcus but the lavage fluid was positive for toxoplasma DNA by

PCR and toxoplasma was grown in tissue culture. An endomyo-cardial biopsy did not show any abnormalities.

Question

1. What is the differential diagnosis?
2. What treatment would you suggest?

Answers

1. Cardiomyopathy with left ventricular failure can be caused by HIV myocarditis, opportunistic infection, nutritional defi-ciencies such as selenium, and drugs such as cocaine.
2. Pyrimethamine and clindamycin.

Comment

AZT has not been proven to cause cardiomyopathy and in fact the relatively low MCV of this patient suggested that he was not complying with AZT at all. Among the opportunistic infections that can produce this picture are EBV, CMV, cryptococcosis and toxoplasmosis. Coxsackievirus can produce myocarditis in the AIDS population just as in the non-AIDS population. In this case, given the documented reactivation of pulmonary toxoplas-mosis, the diagnosis is almost certainly that of toxoplasma myo-carditis.

Echocardiography has shown myocardial dysfunction in a large number of patients with HIV disease and around 10% will have left ventricular dilatation or decreased contractility. How-ever, congestive cardiac failure is very rare. Toxoplasma has been described as a cause of cardiac disease in the immuno-compromised population, producing pericarditis, tamponade, ECG abnormalities, cardiomegaly and congestive cardiac fail-ure. Cardiac involvement with toxoplasma is well described in AIDS and there is evidence that treatment with pyrimethamine and clindamycin has been effective. There was no evidence of cerebral toxoplasmosis in this case, but even so there does seem to have been a cardiopulmonary reactivation and in view of the raised creatine kinase, involvement of skeletal muscles also. A negative endomyocardial biopsy is of no value and autopsy studies on immunocompetent patients with lymphocytic myocarditis have shown such a high rate of false negative results that only a positive biopsy result should be considered useful. The negative IgM for toxoplasma is typical of reactivation disease and the level of toxoplasma IgG can rise during the course of the illness but is not a definite indicator of reactivation. Toxoplasma can be grown in tissue culture but it presents a clinical hazard to laboratory staff and should only be attempted in reference centres.

This patient had hepatosplenomegaly as a result of congestive cardiac failure but fever and hepatosplenomegaly should always suggest the possibility of lymphoma, disseminated CMV infection and disseminated mycobacterium avium intracellulare infection. Cryptococcus can cause myocarditis and muscle tenderness as well as a variety of chest X-ray shadows, but cryptococcus was eliminated in this case by a negative test for cryptococcal antigen in the blood and no growth of cryptococcus in the broncho–alveolar lavage or blood cultures.

Further reading

CALABRESE, L. H., PROFFITT, M. R., YEN-LIEBERMAN, B. *et al.* (1987) Congestive cardiomyopathy and illness related to the acquired immune deficiency syndrome (AIDS) associated with isolation of retrovirus from myocardium. *Ann. Intern. Med.*, **107**, 691–692.

Case 25 An elderly man with bone marrow histiocytosis

A 75-year-old man was referred to hospital by his family practitioner with a 2-week history of high fevers, night sweats and malaise. The present illness appeared suddenly and followed an influenza-like illness some 4 weeks previously. On admission, he appeared pale but otherwise well. There was mild, non-tender hepatosplenomegaly and cervical, axillary and inguinal lymphadenopathy. The peripheral blood showed: Hb 6.4 g/dl, platelets 18×10^9/l, WBC 1.7×10^9/l. Bone marrow biopsy and aspirate showed erythroid and myeloid hypoplasia with prominent megakaryocytes and histiocytic hyperplasia. The histiocytes were mature and cytologically benign but showed prominent phagocytosis of erythrocytes and platelets (haemophagocytosis). A lymph node biopsy showed increased numbers of cytologically benign histiocytes manifesting haemophagocytosis with an intact nodal architecture. The patient made a steady recovery with supportive measures only and the peripheral blood counts were almost normal after a month. His marrow was completely normal 5 months after his presentation to hospital. Viral serology showed a rise of adenovirus complement-fixing antibody from 64 to 1024 between acute and convalescent sera.

Questions

1. What is the likely diagnosis?
2. What is the prognosis?

Answers

1. The major differential diagnosis here is between a malignant histiocytosis and the benign histiocytic proliferation occasionally seen in viral syndromes: the virus - associated haemophagocytic syndrome (VAHS). All of the following suggest the VAHS:
   (i) the antecedent influenzal illness;
   (ii) the marrow and lymph node findings of cytologically benign histiocytosis;
   (iii) the marrow and node findings of marked haemophagocytosis;
   (iv) preservation of the lymph node architecture;
   (v) the benign clinical course and subsequent full recovery;
   (vi) the adenoviral titre rise;
   Although a number of viruses have been associated with the syndrome, a specific virological diagnosis is frequently not made and the clinical criteria are more critical.
2. The prognosis is good and full recovery is the rule. This makes the distinction from malignant syndromes or other processes critical for management.

Further reading

RISDALL, R. J., McKENNA, R. W., NESBIT, M. E. *et al.* (1979) Virus-associated hemophagocytic syndrome. *Cancer,* **44**, 993–1002.

Case 26   Fatigue after acute infection

A 21-year-old girl was seen in the outpatient department complaining of fatigue for the previous 6 months.

She had been a very active sportswoman at school, was now studying law at university where she had been a member of the rowing team, and was keen on amateur dramatics. Her studies had been going well, but 6 months previously she had suffered from sore throat, swollen lymph nodes in the neck and a fever. The illness had been preceded by several days of anorexia, and during the illness she complained of headache and malaise. She consulted her GP at university who found her to have a temperature of 38°C, an exudative pharyngitis and moderately tender posterior and anterior cervical lymph nodes. There was mild tenderness over the right hypochondrium and a throat swab grew Group A beta haemolytic streptococci. She was treated with penicillin and the pharyngitis and fever resolved in 10 days. The lymph nodes remained enlarged for 3 weeks. A full blood count at the time showed a lymphocytosis with cells of abnormal morphology suggestive of infectious mononucleosis. There was a mild neutropenia, thrombocytopenia and a small increase in hepatic transaminases. A monospot test was positive.

Following the resolution of the acute symptoms, she was left with a feeling of pronounced malaise. Her symptoms 6 months later were physical fatigue after exertion, mental fatigue after reading, and wishing to fall asleep in the day even though she had slept all night. She was irritable with her mother at home, not wanting to meet her friends and generally just sitting around all day. Results in the clinic showed normal FBC, urea, electrolytes, liver function tests, thyroid profile, ESR, CRP, rheumatoid factor, antinuclear factor and complement levels.

Questions

1. What is the likely diagnosis?
2. What is the treatment?

Answers

1. Post-glandular fever fatigue.
2. None known. This is a self limiting disease.

Comment

The diagnosis of infectious mononucleosis is not difficult. The combination of fever, pharyngitis and lymphadenopathy together with atypical lymphocytes and a positive monospot test is virtually always due to Epstein–Barr virus (EBV) and no further tests are required. Some patients, especially children, may be monospot negative or may not show atypical lymphocytosis. If there is a suspicion, EBV-specific antibodies should be sought. Most adults with monospot spot-negative mononucleosis are affected with cytomegalovirus, and the presentation is dominated by fever and malaise rather than by pharyngitis and lymphadenopathy.

Severe pharyngitis can be produced by other viruses or by Group A beta haemolytic streptococci. Beta haemolytic streptococci can be isolated in 30% of glandular fever cases, and such isolation does not exclude infectious mononucleosis. Atypical lymphocytosis can be seen in rubella, hepatitis, toxoplasmosis and drug reactions, and these other possibilities should be explored if the monospot is negative.

The use of steroids in infectious mononucleosis is limited to cases of airway obstruction, haemolytic anaemia or thrombocytopenia. Otherwise, the treatment is rest and paracetamol, and patients should be advised to avoid contact sports for the subsequent 2 months because of the very rare possibility of splenic rupture. Other complications of EBV infection are neurological (encephalitis, mononeuritis multiplex, transverse myelitis), and cardiac (pericarditis, myocarditis). This patient shows a very frequent complication, namely post-viral fatigue; interestingly, this seems to affect those without very high fevers or severe pharyngitis at the original illness.

In a patient with fatigue of long duration and normal physical examination, only a few blood tests need to be performed. These are full blood count, urea, electrolytes, liver function tests, calcium, phosphate, erythrocyte sedimentation rate, C-reactive protein, thyroid function tests and a rheumatology screen. A chest X-ray and ECG are sometimes performed and if all these tests are negative, further investigations are very rarely helpful.

There is certainly a fatigue syndrome that follows glandular fever. The sufferers are mainly from socioeconomic groups 1 and 2 and in their early twenties, perhaps because persons from lower social-economic classes have EBV infections in childhood. The fatigue syndrome comprises physical fatigue (especially after exertion), mental fatigue, hypersomnia, motor retardation, poor concentration, loss of pleasure in usual activities, irritability and, at the onset of illness, anorexia.

A number of patients present to infectious diseases clinics complaining of very long-standing fatigue, sometimes after a presumed viral illness. These are often white women of between 30 and 40 years of age with an average duration of symptoms of 5 years. Physical examination and laboratory investigations are usually normal, and this group has been classified as having chronic fatigue syndrome with symptoms of mental fatigue, joint pains, muscle pains, poor concentration, malaise after effort and sleep disturbance. There is no consistent evidence of a single disease process or evidence of viral, immunological, muscular or neurological causes for this collection of symptoms. Many in this group suffer from fibromyalgia, a rheumatological condition characterised by tender nodules in the neck, over the scapulae, the hips and the lower back. It is associated with irritable bowel syndrome and sometimes depression. Fibromyalgia is thought to be a consequence of sleep disturbance, and can be reproduced in normal volunteers by sleep deprivation. Patients with very long-standing fatigue most often complain of insomnia and muscle pains, whereas those with post-viral fatigue do not complain of muscle pains and have hypersomnia.

Patients with very long-standing fatigue can display marked psychiatric problems. Around half of these patients suffer from a major depressive illness and around 10% from panic disorder. Around 10% suffer from somatization disorder, which is the presentation of psychological distress with multiple somatic symptoms without objective medical findings. Patients with somatization disorder travel from doctor to doctor and generate investigation costs that may be six times higher than other patients. Such patients can take up half the time of primary care physicians even though they form less than 1% of the population.

Caution should be used in making the diagnosis of somatization, as patients with syphilis, SLE, multiple sclerosis, porphyria and HIV infection can present in very bizarre ways. It is best to use a four-step screening cluster for somatization disorder.

1. Unless there is a current or past history of medically unexplained pain in at least four different parts of the body, the diagnosis is excluded.
2. Unless two or more gastrointestinal symptoms other than pain (e.g. nausea, vomiting, diarrhoea, food intolerance) are

reported, the diagnosis is excluded.
3. At least one sexual reproductive symptom is required for diagnosis.
4. At least one conversion symptom (pseudoneurological) is required.

The disease should have an onset before the age of 30 years and duration of several years before a diagnosis is considered.

Whereas patients with post-viral fatigue will suffer from sleepiness and depression, patients with somatization disorder will absolutely deny any psychiatric symptoms and focus on a vast array of physical complaints.

There is no proven treatment for post-viral fatigue, or chronic fatigue syndrome.

Fibromyalgia should be treated with low doses of amitryptiline at night, together with supervised graded exercise.

Evaluation of patients with very prolonged fatigue should include psychiatric screening, especially for major depressive illness, and a search for primary sleep disorders such as sleep apnoea. Patients with sleep apnoea or periodic leg movement disorder can present with features indistinguishable from chronic fatigue syndrome and primary sleep disorders should be suspected in any patient who reports an overwhelming urge to sleep during the day, especially if the urge is irresistible.

Further reading

LLEWELYN, M. B. (1996) Assessing the fatigued patient. *British Journal of Hospital Medicine*, **55**, 125–129.

Case 27   Unexpected deterioration in cystic fibrosis

A 12-year-old boy with cystic fibrosis was admitted to a cystic fibrosis ward on the paediatric wing of a general hospital suffering from an acute lower respiratory tract infection. Initial therapy with intravenous flucloxacillin and gentamicin failed to produce any response after 24 h, by which time a light growth of a pseudomonas-like organism was seen on selective media.

Two months prior to admission the patient had been on a camping trip with patients with cystic fibrosis in North America. Pulmonary function appeared to have deteriorated unexpectedly and progressively following this trip.

Questions

1. What is the major concern?
2. What should be the empirical cover whilst awaiting sensitivities?
3. What is the prognosis?
4. What are the infection control issues/in hospital and in the community?

Answers

1. The major concern is that the patient is now infected with *Burkholderia (Pseudomonas) cepacia* acquired from another patient during the North American camping trip.
2. *B. cepacia* is multiresistant but usually retains sensitivity to ceftazidime and this agent is a good choice in high doses for empirical therapy. In less acute situations, i.e. for patients who are colonized, some advocate a cessation of all antibiotics in the hope that *P. aeruginosa* will overgrow and possibly eradicate *B. cepacia*. Note that the organism grows slowly and selective plates should be held for 72 h with re-incubation.
3. For reasons which are not fully understood, pulmonary function begins to deteriorate following acquisition of this organism and may lead to earlier mortality. Unlike the case with *P. aeruginosa*, a mechanism for lung damage cannot be linked with identifiable virulence factors in *B. cepacia*.
4. Both community and nosocomial spread of this organism amongst patients with cystic fibrosis have been documented. Guidelines are available from the Cystic Fibrosis Society (UK) for the control of spread in both environments. Patients with the organism should not have close contact with non-colonized patients, as may occur for example, during camping trips. In hospital, respiratory precautions or its equivalent e.g. separate wards for colonized and non-colonized patients, must be seriously considered with due sensitivity to the social needs of the patients.

Further reading

WALTERS, S. and SMITH, E.G. (1993) Pseudomonas cepacia in cystic fibrosis: transmissibility and its implications. *Lancet*, **343**, 3–4.

Case 28 Fever and chest pain following aortic valve replacement

C.D. had been a hard-working farmer all his life, and had never troubled his general practitioner. Encouraged to go for health screening by his wife, he was noted to have a murmur of aortic regurgitation by his doctor. A subsequent chest X-ray showed enlargement of the heart and he was referred for a cardiology opinion following which (6 months later) the aortic valve was replaced by a Carpentier–Edwards prosthesis.

However, 2 weeks after leaving hospital he was readmitted because he had developed chills, left-sided chest pain and some shortness of breath on climbing stairs.

There was no relevant family history and he was taking a combination tablet of 40 mg of frusemide and 5 mg of amiloride a day. There was no history of tuberculosis.

On examination, temperature was 38°C, pulse 90/minute regular, BP 130/80 mmHg. He appeared comfortable, with no clubbing and the venous pressure was not raised. There was dullness to percussion and absence of breath sounds at the left lung base. A systolic murmur was heard over the aortic area, but no diastolic murmur or friction rub. Abdominal examination was normal, and no abnormality was found in the central nervous system. Dipstick testing of urine was normal.

Laboratory investigations showed: Hb 11.0 g/dl, WBC 4.0×10^9/l (80% neutrophils), MCV 90 fl, platelets 360×10^9/l, ESR 108 mm/h. Clotting screen was normal, as were urea, electrolytes, liver function tests, calcium and phosphate. ECG showed sinus rhythm at 100/min and there was left axis deviation consistent with previous aortic regurgitation. A chest X-ray showed the Carpentier–Edwards prosthesis, enlargement of the cardiac shadow and a small left sided pleural effusion. Transthoracic echocardiography showed a normal prosthetic valve and a normal sized left ventricle surrounded by a moderate pericardial effusion. No vegetations were seen on the valve.

Repeated blood cultures were sterile and testing for anti-nuclear factor, rheumatoid factor, RNP and Ro/La antibodies were all negative. The ANCA, and hepatitis A, B, and C serology were negative. Serology for cytomegalovirus and HIV were negative and the angiotensin converting enzyme level was normal. A tuberculin test was negative and serology for Brucella, Q fever and psittacosis were all negative. A CT scan of the chest did not demonstrate any lung or mediastinal pathology.

Question

1. Name the two most likely diagnoses?
2. What are the next two investigations you would performed?

Answers

1. a. Post-pericardiotomy syndrome;
   b. Endocarditis.
2. Aspiration of pericardial fluid for microscopy and culture
   Trans-oesophageal echocardiography.

Comment

This man developed a fever 2 weeks after aortic valve replacement, accompanied by pericardial and pleural effusions. The pericardial effusion is not producing a tamponade as the jugular venous pressure is not raised and no paradoxical pulse is reported. Pericarditis of any cause usually gives rise to a small left-sided pleural effusion, and the differential diagnosis should focus on the pericardial fluid. Table 1 lists the causes of a pericardial fluid collection after open heart surgery.

Table 1: Causes of pericarditis after open heart surgery

Post-operative haematoma
Bacterial endocarditis
Post-pericardiotomy syndrome
Talc or cellulose paper granulomas

Rarer causes would include those not necessarily related to surgery, such as systemic lupus erythematosus, systemic vasculitis, rheumatoid arthritis and tuberculosis. Many of these conditions have been excluded by the diagnostic workup.

The first consideration in a feverish patient with a heart prosthesis is endocarditis. In the year following valve replacement, around 3% will develop a prosthetic valve infection. Most early cases of prosthetic valve endocarditis (PVE) occur in the first 2 months, and therefore are likely to be caused by contamination at surgery. Such early infection is likely to be caused by *Staphylococcus epidermidis*, diphtheroids, Gram-negative rods, candida, enterococci or S*taph. aureus*. These early infections can cause severe damage to the valve by invading the surrounding myocardium, and the mycocardium can be penetrated resulting in pericarditis. Tracking of the infection can also produce conduction changes detectable on ECG. Clinically, dehiscence of the valve caused by infection may be associated with a diastolic murmur. Infected prosthetic valves often require surgical intervention and infection should be assiduously sought. Transthoracic echocardiagram at best detects vegetations in 80% of patients and trans-oesophageal echocardiography is preferred.

Blood cultures are usually positive, if four cultures of 20 ml each are taken at intervals of a few hours. Negative cultures might be found in infections with slowly growing bacteria such as haemophilus para-influenzae, brucella or some streptococcal species. Aspergillus endocarditis is virtually never detected by blood culture and psittacosis and Q fever require serology for diagnosis. If the valve were to be infected, mortality can be as high as 50%. In this case, trans-oesophageal echocardiogram was normal and multiple blood cultures and serology were negative.

Another possible disease to consider is tuberculosis and it is worth noting that tuberculous pericarditis is often accompanied by a negative tuberculin test. Pericardial biopsy might be needed to establish this diagnosis.

Post-pericardiotomy syndrome appears to be an auto-immune reaction following cardiac surgery. It develops in 50% of patients who have had open heart surgery and is often accompanied by a left-sided lymphocytic pleural effusion. It seems more common with patients with aortic rather than mitral valve replacement and can result in thickening of the pericardium and encapsulation of fluid by adhesions.

The foreign body granulomatous reaction to talc from gloves has been largely dealt with by eliminating irritating materials and careful glove washing, but cellulose from the paper clothing worn in theatre has been reported to produce peritoneal granu-lomas. A further cause of fever after cardiac by-pass is 'post-per-fusion' syndrome comprising fever, atypical lymphocytosis and splenomegaly. However, this does not produce a pericarditis.

The usual management would be to aspirate the pericardial fluid for culture, and if this were negative to prescribe indo-methacin for presumed post-pericardiotomy syndrome. If the fever persisted, then operative pericardial drainage and pericardial biopsy might be required.

Further reading

BRAIMBRIDGE, M. V. and EYKYN, S. J. (1987) Prosthetic valve endocarditis. *J. Antimicrob. Chemother.*, **20** (Supplement A), 173.

Case 29   Acute red eye in an ophthalmologist

A consultant ophthalmologist developed an acute red eye with pre-auricular lymphadenopathy. The next day his registrar was also afflicted, as were two other consultants and four patients who had been recently seen in the ophthalmology outpatients. The syndrome appeared to be a bilateral follicular conjunctivi-tis with mild fever and headache but no respiratory symptoms. Two of the patients subsequently reported that other family members developed red eyes.

Questions

1. What is the likely cause of this suspected outbreak of kerato-conjunctivitis?
2. How is it spread?
3. How is the diagnosis confirmed?
4. What is the clinical course?

Answers

1. The likely cause is an adenovirus of type 8, 11,19 or 37. This is

consistent with the clinical presentation and observed spread both in the outpatients' department and in the patients' homes.

2. In the hospital setting the most common mode of transmission is ocular examination by medical staff where virus is transferred to the patient by hands or contaminated instruments such as tonometers. Containment requires strict adherence to handwashing, tonometer and environmental decontamination and in some instances, closure of the ophthalmology outpatient suite for a short period for thorough cleaning. In the home setting, transmission is generally by shared towels and hand-to-hand.

3. The diagnosis can be strongly suspected on clinical criteria but confirmation requires conjunctival scrapings for electron microscopy, immunofluorescent detection of viral antigens or, viral isolation in cell culture. Serology is a useful adjunct and should demonstate a four-fold rise in group specific complement fixing antibodies. Further serological tests for neutralizing and haemaglutination-inhibiting antibodies are type specific. Virus can be isolated for up to 9 days after the onset of symptoms and can be grouped and specifically serotyped.

4. The conjunctivitis may last 1–4 weeks, giving way to keratitis with a severe foreign-body sensation, photophobia and lacrimation. Close ophthalmic follow-up is required but there is no specific antiviral treatment.

Comment

Epidemic adenoviral keratoconjunctivitis in adults was first described in 1955 in shipyard workers who had sustained minor trauma to the eyes. Community outbreaks are not infrequent and may in fact be the source of secondary hospital spread from staff or patients. The incubation period is 7–10 days and clinical features include pharyngitis, preauricular lymphadenopathy and follicular conjunctivitis. Whilst symptoms can be severe and distressing, the disease is usually self-limiting and only rarely causes long-term corneal changes and visual impairment.

Further reading

TULLO, A. B. and HIGGINS, P. G. (1980) An outbreak of adenovirus type 14 conjunctivitis. *Br. J. Ophthalmol.*, **64**, 489.

Case 30   A human bite

A 28-year-old woman sustained a bite to her right hand from her male partner during a serious domestic argument. No immediate care was given to the wound and she presented to casualty 3 days later with a swollen and painful right hand. On examination, two puncture marks were noted over the hypothenar eminence with surrounding swelling and erythema. She confirmed that the bite was from her partner and not caused by their two cats. A swab of serosanguinous exudate from one of the punctures was sent to the microbiology department for bacterial culture and she was admitted to hospital for intravenous antibiotics. Cultures subsequently grew smooth grey colonies on sheep blood agar after 1 day of incubation in air plus CO_2 at $35°C$. The organism was a Gram-negative rod that was oxidase positive and sensitive to penicillin.

Questions

1. What organisms commonly cause human bite infections?
2. What is your choice of empirical antimicrobial treatment?

Answers

1. The organisms causing human bite infections are those which normally or occasionally colonize the mouth. In settings where deep infection of bone has also occurred, biopsies have grown mixed cultures including *Eikenella corrodens*, α and β-haemolytic streptococci, *Staphylococcus aureus*, coagulase-negative staphylococci, enteric Gram-negative bacilli and obligate anaerobes such as *Peptostreptococcus* sp. and oral *Bacteroides* sp. In more superficial infections, single isolates or combinations of those mentioned may be found. The organism in this case was *Pasteurella multocida* which is part of the normal oral flora of cats and dogs and associated with bites from these animals. Humans who have close contact with these animals such as kissing may also harbour the organism in the mouth and this is the probable explanation for such isolation in this case.
2. Therapy includes surgical drainage where necessary and

appropriate antimicrobial selection. Empirical antimicrobial therapy should be broad enough to cover the likely causative organisms including penicillinase-producing strains. In this regard co-amoxiclav would be suitable and allows for intravenous therapy and follow-on oral administration. This is a particularly important consideration with the prolonged treatment required for any associated osteomyelitis.

Comment

Human bites can occur anywhere on the body but bites to the hand are most frequent and are more likely to become infected.

Further reading

BROOK, I. (1987) Microbiology of human and animal bite wounds in children. *Pediatr. Infect. Dis.*, **6**, 29–32.

GOLDSTEIN, E. J. C., BARONE, M., MILLER, T. A. (1983) *Eikenella corrodens* in hand infections. *J. Hand Surg*, **8**, 563–567.

Case 31   Hepatic granulomas

A 72-year-old woman was admitted for investigation of fatigue and pyrexia. She had suffered from intermittent fevers for around 2 months, and over that period had become anorexic. She reported no diarrhoea, passage of blood or abdominal pain. She had been taking allopurinol for gout for the previous 6 months and she was not taking HRT. The onset of illness had been gradual; she had never been abroad and had no pets including birds. She had not visited farms and there was no previous history of tuberculosis. She had never had blood transfusions.

On examination, temperature was 37.8°C, pulse 80/min and BP 140/90 mmHg. Examination of the chest and abdomen were normal and the central nervous system was intact.

Investigation showed Hb 10.5 g/dl, MCV 88 fl, WBC $7.4 \times 10^9/l$, ESR 120 mm/h, AST 354 IU/l (10–35) Gamma-glutamyl transpeptidase, alkaline phosphatase, bilirubin, creatinine and creatine phosphokinase were all normal. Tests for cryoglobulins, rheumatoid factor, antimitochondrial antibodies and antinuclear antibodies were negative.

C3 and C4 levels in the serum were normal and tests for HIV, syphilis and hepatitis A, B and C were negative. Standard and mycobacterial cultures of blood and urine were negative after prolonged incubation. A tuberculin test (10 UPPD) was negative; and serology was negative for *Toxoplasma gondii*, brucella, and toxocara. There was evidence of previous CMV and EBV infection but no acute antibody response.

A chest X-ray and ultra-sound scan of the abdomen were normal and CT examination of the abdomen and thorax was negative. Slit-lamp examination of the eyes was normal.

Percutaneous liver biopsy revealed preservation of architecture, with a moderate portal and lobular infiltrate by lymphohistiocytic inflammatory cells, prominent Kupffer cells, focal liver cell necrosis and three epithelial non-caseating granulomas. Ziehl–Neelsen stain for acid-fast bacilli of the biopsy was negative, and there was no response to 1 month of empirical anti-tuberculous chemotherapy on the ward.

Questions

1. What should be the next step?
2. What should be the next treatment?

Answers

1. A trial of stopping allopurinol.
2. Prednisolone.

Comment

Many infectious and non-infectious diseases can produce hepatic granulomas and when they are found there must be a structured approach to differential diagnosis. In tertiary centres, up to 50% of cases will eventually be classified as 'idiopathic' and this is a diagnosis of exclusion.

Table 1 shows the infectious causes of hepatic granulomas.

Table 1: Infectious causes of hepatic granulomas

Bacterial causes
Mycobacteria (tuberculous, non-tuberculous, BCG immunotherapy)
Lepromatous leprosy
Brucella abortus
Cat scratch disease
Listeriosis
Melioidosis
Yersinia enterocolitica

Fungal causes
Candidiasis
Histoplasmosis
Coccidioidomycosis

Viral causes
Cytomegalovirus
Epstein–Barr virus
Viral hepatitis

Rickettsial causes
Q fever

Spirochaetal causes
Syphilis

Parasitic causes
Schistosomiasis
Toxocariasis

This list of infectious causes is still dominated by tuberculosis, and this accounts for around 10% of cases of hepatic granulomas. Tuberculosis ranks second only to sarcoidosis as a cause of non-caseating granulomas of the liver, and in miliary tuberculosis at least 90% of patients will have hepatic granulomas. *M. tuberculosis* may be demonstrated by staining and culture of the biopsy. Instillation of BCG into the bladder as a treatment for bladder cancer can lead to hepatic granulomas. In lepromatous leprosy, Kupffer cells are teeming with bacilli. Brucellosis has been associated with hepatic granulomas, especially *Brucella abortus*. *Brucella suis* and *melitensis* often produce less clear hepatic changes.

An uncommon cause of hepatic granulomas is cat-scratch disease, especially in children. Cat-scratch disease can also cause splenic granulomas and although these lesions usually disappear spontaneously in 1–5 months, the granulomas can later calcify in fine or coarse patterns. Cat-scratch fever can present as a fever of unknown origin and often multiple hypodense lesions may be apparent on ultrasound or CT examination of the liver. The diagnosis can be confirmed by immunoassay for *Bartonella hensalae* or PCR for *B. hensalae* in tissue specimens. Also, the organisms may be visualized in biopsies using the Warthin–Starry stain. Peripheral lymphadenopathy may be completely absent in some of these cases.

The granulomas of Schistosoma mansoni and visceral larva migrans may be the result of egg deposition producing a foreign body reaction, as well as a specific immune response.

Coxiella burnetti, which causes Q fever, can be associated with granulomatous hepatitis and unlike other rickettsioses it does not cause a skin rash. Q fever can present in a manner identical to viral hepatitis and can lead to a prolonged febrile illness, sometimes with acute respiratory involvement. Bone marrow examination may also reveal granulomas and *C. burnetti* antibodies should be sought in cases of granulomatous hepatitis.

Table 2 shows non-infectious causes of hepatic granulomas.

Table 2: Non-infectious causes of hepatic granulomas

Sarcoidosis
Hypersensitivity reactions (e.g. erythema nodosum, drugs)
Primary liver disease (especially primary biliary cirrhosis)
Neoplasms (especially Hodgkin's)
Immune deficiency (chronic granulomatous disease and hypogamma-globulinaemia)
Temporal arteritis
Ulcerative colitis and Crohn's disease
Idiopathic hepatic granulomas

This was a case of temporal arteritis, or giant cell arteritis, and the diagnosis was supported by a temporal artery biopsy. There were no visual signs, jaw claudication or temporal artery tenderness, and the patient made a good response to steroids. Abnormal liver function tests are well known in giant cell arteritis, and commonly only the alkaline phosphatase is raised. Usually, liver biopsy in giant cell arteritis shows no abnormalities but granulomas have been well described in the literature.

When major causes of granulomas such as tuberculosis and sarcoidosis have been excluded, it would appear reasonable to start a patient over 50 years old on an empirical course of steroids as often a dramatic response is seen. Because of the risk of occult tuberculosis, patients are often given antituberculous therapy in the first instance, as administering steroids in a case of TB could be potentially catastrophic.

In cases of hepatic granulomata, hypersensitivity to drugs is a common forgotten cause, and drugs especially likely to produce this include allopurinol, augmentin, carbamazepine and dapsone.

Further reading

ZOUTMAN, D. E., RALPH, E. D. and FREI, J. V. (1991) Granulomatous hepatitis and fever of unknown origin. An 11-yr experience of 23 cases with three years' follow-up. *J. Clin. Gastroenterol.*, **13**, 69–73.

Case 32   A young woman with vaginal discharge

A 26-year-old female presented to her family practitioner with a persistent vaginal discharge. She was sexually active but claimed to have had a monogamous relationship with her boyfriend of 8 months. He was apparently well with no urethral discharge or dysuria. A screen for gonorrhoea, chlamydia and trichomonas was negative and there were no relevant laboratory data to suggest candidal vaginitis. However, the laboratory did report a light growth of *Gardnerella vaginalis.*

Questions

1. Is this bacterial vaginosis and how is this diagnosis best established?
2. Is it sexually transmitted?
3. What is the treatment?

Answers

1. The vogue for culturing *G. vaginalis* as a means of diagnosing bacterial vaginosis has now passed, since up to 20% of young sexually active women may harbour the organism in the lower genital tract without evidence of disease. Any three of the following signs strongly support the diagnosis:
   (i) a thin, homogeneous, white, adherent discharge;
   (ii) vaginal pH greater than 4.5;

   (iii) the presence of an amine odour with the addition of 10% KOH (positive 'whiff' test).

   (iv) the presence of 'clue cells' (epithelial cells studded with bacteria) seen on wet mount or Gram-stain preparations of vaginal secretions.

2. Bacterial vaginosis is essentially a non-inflammatory syndrome caused by overgrowth of normal anaerobes (*Bacteroides, Peptococcus, Eubacterium, Bifidobacterium* and *Mobiluncus*) and facultative anaerobes (*G. vaginalis, S. viridans*) in the lower genital tract. An associated decrease in normal vaginal lactobacilli is also observed. Although classified in textbooks as a sexually transmitted disease the case is far from proven. For example, no male counterpart of the syndrome has been fully described, although *Gardnerella balanitis* may occur. The issue has practical consequences since the label of 'sexually transmitted disease' can have profound psycho-social implications for the patient.

3. Oral metronidazole or intravaginal clindamycin ointment have both been found to be effective, but it may be preferable not to use metronidazole in pregnancy. Co-amoxiclav may be used in pregnancy. The aim of treatment is to relieve symptoms, although some evidence suggests that bacterial vaginosis may predispose to upper genital tract disease, preterm labour and post-Caesarean section endometritis.

Further reading

SPIEGEL, C. A. (1991) Bacterial vaginosis. *Clin. Microbiol. Rev.*, **4**, 485–502.

AMSEL, R., TOTTEN, P. A., SPIEGEL, C. A. *et al* (1983) Non-specific vaginitis: Diagnostic criteria and microbial and epidemiological associations. *Am. J. Med.*, **74**, 14.

ANDRES, F., PARKER, R., HOSEIN, I. and BENRUBI, G. (1992) Clindamycin vaginal cream versus oral metronidazole in the treatment of bacterial vaginosis. *Southern Medical Journal*, **85**, 1077–1080.

Case 33   A child with failure to thrive, recurrent boils and chronic purulent rhinitis

A 2-year-old caucasian boy was on the paediatric ward because of fever of unknown origin. He was the third child of a 30-year-old mother, born normally at term. At the age of 1 he developed a chronic runny nose and impetigo. Chest X-ray and sinus X-ray at that time were both normal, but his mother then began to notice recurrent 'boils' on his face and chest. Later, these appeared around the nose and seemed to improve with antibiotics.

Two weeks prior to admission he had a fever and a large painless lymph node was found by his mother in the left posterior cervical area; following a negative tuberculin test at a BCG clinic he was prescribed flucloxacillin. On admission the lymph node had to be surgically drained because it had become fluctuant. Microscopy of pus from the node showed many neutrophils and Gram-positive cocci in clusters but no acid-fast bacilli or fungal elements.

S. aureus was grown on culture. One week later, whilst still in the ward, a right cervical lymph node was found to be painlessly enlarged, and he was documented to have a fever again.

On examination, his weight was below the 50th percentile, temperature 36.5°C, pulse 130/min. respiratory rate 45/min. Blood pressure was 85 mmHg systolic. A 2.5 cm^3 non-tender lymph node was palpated in the right anterior cervical region but no other lymphadenopathy was found. A repeat tuberculin test was negative; candidal antigen skin test was positive. Chest, abdominal and CNS examinations were normal and there was no skin rash.

Laboratory investigations showed: Hb 11.8 g/dl, WBC 19.6 × 10^9/l (44% neutrophils), platelets 545 × 10^9/l, clotting screen normal, ESR 45 mm/h; urea and electrolytes and liver enzymes were normal. Total IgG levels normal, IgG subclasses 1–4 present, IgA, IgM, and IgE levels normal. C3 and C4 levels and total haemolytic complement were normal. Blood and urine cultures were sterile and an HIV antibody test was negative.

A chest X-ray and ultrasound of the abdomen were normal. Flucloxacillin was given intravenously.

Questions

1. What is the likely diagnosis?
2. What test would you perform to confirm this?

Answers

1. Chronic granulomatous disease.
2. The nitroblue tetrazolium test.

Comment

This child is clearly unwell with failure to thrive, recurrent boils, impetigo, purulent rhinitis and a suppurative lymphadenitis.

The history is suggestive of an immune deficiency, either primary or secondary. Common causes of secondary immunodeficiency would be nephrotic syndrome, HIV infection, splenic dysfunction, steroids and intercurrent malignancy. In this case the HIV antibody test was negative, there was no proteinuria and splenic dysfunction is unlikely, as this is usually manifested by infection with encapsulated bacteria such as *Strep. pneumoniae, Haemophilus influenzae* and *Neisseria meningitidis.*

Primary immune disorders include those affecting complement, antibody production, T cell number or function and the phagocytic dysfunction diseases. In this case, antibody levels are normal, there is a normal delayed skin response to candida antigens, the complement system is normal and there appears to be a normal array of white cells in the blood.

One aspect of immunity not tested here is the assessment of phagocytic function. Phagocytic dysfunction can give rise to skin abscesses, lymphadenitis, and bone and liver abscesses. The usual infecting organism is *Staphylococcus aureus.*

Examples of phagocytic defects are Job's syndrome (characterized by very high IgE levels, impaired chemotaxis of neutrophils, pneumonia and cold abscesses) and leucocyte adhesion molecule deficiencies (producing infections in the skin and middle ear, a white cell count of up to 50 000 in the blood and, impaired pus formation). Neither of these diseases seems likely as the IgE level and total white cell count are normal.

This child is suffering from chronic granulomutous disease with yet another bacterial lymph node infection. Confirmation is with the nitroblue tetrazolium (NBT) dye reduction test in which neutrophils are stimulated with yeast particles in the presence of NBT. Superoxide produced by normal neutrophils reduces yellow NBT dye to a deep blue pigment which can be seen by microscopy. In this case blue dye formation was severely impaired although the yeast particles were ingested normally. In chronic granulomatous disease, there is a defect in one of the four protein components of NADPH oxidase caused by point mutations in the relevant genes. When NADPH oxidase is assembled, there is reduction of molecular oxygen which provides superoxide.

The disease is characterized by necrotizing granulomatous inflammation occurring in the skin, lymph nodes, lung, liver and other sites, because there is ineffective killing of a number of bacteria and fungi, especially *Staph. aureus* and *Enterobacter* sp; the most common fungal infections are caused by aspergillus which can affect the brain and bones.

After surgical drainage of infected areas, prolonged antibiotic therapy must be administered.

General management includes counselling the patient to avoid exposure to aspergillus, for example in freshly cut grass. Interferon gamma produces a 67% reduction in serious infections requiring antibiotics, and some patients are maintained on prophylactic interferon gamma given three times a week as well as prophylactic antibiotics. Occasionally patients are maintained on prophylactic itraconazole to prevent infection with aspergillus. Improved therapy has meant that many of these patients can live into middle age.

Further reading

GALLIN, J. I. and MALECH, H. L. (1990) Update on chronic granulomatous diseases of childhood: Immunotherapy and potential for gene therapy. *JAMA*, **263**, 1533.

Case 34 A young West Indian woman with infertility and possible chronic pelvic infection

A 28-year-old woman from Trinidad presented for evaluation of infertility. Ten years previously she had had a D & C performed for persistent menorrhagia. Over the ensuing years she had had recurrent episodes of lower abdominal pain with associated fevers to 39°C and a heavy yellowish vaginal discharge. Laboratory investigation revealed trichomonas at one point which responded to a course of metronidazole. Repeated courses of antimicrobial therapy for presumed pelvic inflammatory disease were unsuccessful. A hysterosalpingogram showed a normal uterine fundus and bilateral obstruction of the Fallopian tubes. A recent endometrial biopsy was reported as showing granulomatous inflammation. Physical examination was essentially normal apart from mild right lower quadrant pain.

Questions

1. What disease is suggested by the data presented?
2. How does it arise?
3. Is it notifiable?
4. What is the prognosis?

Answers

1. The features described suggest pelvic tuberculosis which usually presents with infertility. The menstrual irregularities and lack of response of presumed pelvic inflammatory disease to antimicrobial therapy are also suggestive in the right epidemiological setting. The granulomatous inflammation seen on the endometrial biopsy is only infrequently seen. A stain for acid-fast bacilli must be done and samples submitted for mycobacterial culture.
2. Pelvic tuberculosis arises by haematogenous seeding of the endosalpinx from a pulmonary focus (which may not be clinically apparent).
3. All forms of tuberculosis are notifiable. It is important to bear in mind that notification is required not just on laboratory confirmation but also on clinical suspicion especially in the case of pulmonary tuberculosis.
4. The response to chemotherapy is excellent but residual tubal fibrosis may still cause infertility or predispose to ectopic pregnancy.

Further reading

CARTER, J. R. (1990) Unusual presentations of genital tract tuberculosis. *Int. J. Gynecol. Obstet.*, **33**, 171–176.

Case 35   A boy with cellulitis of the foot

A 12-year-old boy sustained a nail puncture through his trainers whilst out running. He presented to the A & E department of a local hospital where the lesion was noted to be close to the right great toe on the plantar aspect but felt to be superficial. After local cleaning, topical antiseptics were applied and he was sent home with a 7-day course of oral co-amoxiclav (amoxycillin-clavulanate). He had recently received a tetanus booster vaccine and no further management was felt to be required in this regard. After 4 days, pain and tenderness developed at the puncture site. He did not re-present until cellulitis had developed some 2 weeks after first being seen.

Questions

1. What is the most serious potential diagnosis and what pathogen must be considered?
2. What is the treatment?

Answers

1. The most serious diagnosis to be entertained is osteochondritis of the foot from *Pseudomonas aeruginosa* – in this case possibly affecting the first metacarpophalangeal joint. The infection may be primary in that the joint may have been involved in the initial puncture with inoculation of the organism or could result from soft tissue cellulitis spreading deeper. The association with trainers (sneakers) probably reflects the increased finding of this organism in such footwear because of the moist environment. This has led to the occasional use of the term 'sneaker osteomyelitis'.
2. The treatment is both surgical and medical. Surgical debridement is performed urgently with exploration and drainage; necrotic tissue removed must be submitted for Gram-staining and culture. Empirical antimicrobial treatment is with high dose anti-pseudomonal agents such as ciprofloxacin, imipenem or ceftazidime (co-amoxiclav has no anti-pseudomonal activity). The diagnosis is commonly confirmed by growth of the organism from the tissue submitted. Treatment

is usually continued for 4–6 weeks, although shorter courses may suffice.

Comment

Pseudomonas infections of bones and joints are not uncommon and arise by both haemotogenous seeding and spread from a contiguous focus. Blood borne infections of the sternoclavicular and sacroiliac joints are particularly associated with IV drug users. Pseudomonas osteochondritis was first described following puncture wounds to the foot in children but can occur in any age group. A biphasic illness with initial improvement followed by recurrence of symptoms is typical. Systemic features are not usually present even though the condition may be so locally destructive.

In antimicrobial therapeutics it is quite common on the wards to hear of this or that agent 'covering' a number of organisms. There are two caveats to this approach which must be remembered. First, 'cover' does not mean 'optimal'. Whilst a given agent may have sufficient activity against a number of organisms in a given clinical situation to be used for empirical management, therapy must be modified to include an optimal agent or combination of agents as the diagnosis becomes more certain. Secondly, in the rush to name the myriad organisms 'covered', critical ones against which an agent has no significant activity are missed. This is the concept of the microbial 'therapeutic hole'. As an example, recall the following: no cephalosporin antibiotic has any activity against MRSA, enterococci or listeria; very few have anti-pseudomonal or anti-anaerobic activities; care must be exercised in the use of cephalosporins against *Enterobacter* sp. because of possible emergence of resistance on therapy (by selection of derepressed mutants producing high levels of cephalosporinase).

Further reading

JACOBS, R. F., McCARTHY, R. E. and ELSER, J. M. (1989) *Pseudomonas* osteochondritis complicating puncture wounds of the foot in children: a 10-year evaluation. *J. Infect. Dis.*, **160**, 657–661.

FISHER, M. C., GOLDSMITH, J. F. and GILLIGAN, P. H. (1985) Sneakers as a source of *Pseudomonas aeruginosa* in children with osteomyelitis following puncture wounds. *J. Pediatr.*, **106**, 607–609.

CHOW, J. W., FINE, M. J., SCHLOES, D. M. *et al.* (1991) Enterobacter bacteremia: clinical features and emergence of antibiotic resistance during therapy. *Ann. Int. Med.*, **115**, 585–590

Case 36 An abnormal chest X-ray after bone marrow transplantation

A 60-year-old man was admitted to the haematology ward, having suffered from relapsed diffuse large cell lymphoma. It was decided to treat him with an autologous bone marrow transplant.

The conditioning regimen included carmustine, etoposide and cytarabine and was started 6 days prior to transplant.

Two days prior to the transplant he started to become short of breath. A chest X-ray showed an increase in pulmonary vascular markings but an echocardiogram was normal.

Autologous marrow (2×10^8 cells/kg, cryopreserved in 10% DMSO) was infused through a central venous catheter. Shortly after infusion, the patient became acutely short of breath and blood gases showed a pO_2 of 40 mm Hg on air. His weight was 4 kg over baseline, and intravenous frusemide was given with improvement. After the marrow infusion, the serum LDH rose to 1165 IU/l (80–225) and remained high.

On the day after transplant, fever was noted and vancomycin, piperacillin and gentamicin were started empirically. Blood cultures subsequently grew *Klebsiella pneumoniae*, sensitive to piperacillin and gentamicin.

On the ninth day after transplant the fever returned and amphotericin B was added.

The neutrophil count by day 15 was 0.8×10^9/l, supported by G-CSF.

On day 16 the patient developed severe shortness of breath and haemoptysis. A chest X-ray showed bilateral diffuse alveolar infiltrates and fibreoptic bronchoscopy with bronchoalveolar lavage found haemorrhagic fluid with persistently blood stained aliquots being obtained. A coagulation screen was normal, platelet count 40×10^9/l, and culture and microscopy of the lavage fluid was negative.

Question

1. What is the probable diagnosis?

Answer

1. Diffuse alveolar haemorrhage (DAH).

Comment

When called to see patients with suspected infections, one should be aware of non-infectious illnesses that can occur in particular settings. This is especially true in the case of transplantation medicine.

The syndrome of diffuse alveolar haemorrhage has been described since 1989 in patients undergoing autologous bone marrow transplantation (BMT). It affects 10–20% of autologous BMT patients and is fatal in around half the cases. It is characterized by shortness of breath, fever, cough, mucositis, low pO_2 and a chest X-ray that shows diffuse infiltrates. Bronchoalveolar lavage fluid can become bloodier with each aliquot recovered. Symptoms usually occur 12 days after marrow infusion, when the neutrophil count starts to recover. The rise in serum LDH is a particularly common finding in DAH.

Lung complications are a major cause of morbidity and mortality in patients undergoing any form of transplantation, and can be non-infectious or non-infectious in origin (Table 1).

Table 1: **Causes of lung problems following organ transplantation**

Infectious complications
CMV pneumonia
Pneumocystis pneumonia
Aspergillus
Candida
Nocardia
Legionella

Non-infectious complications in various forms of organ transplantation
Bone marrow – drugs, radiation, DAH, bronchiolitis obliterans
Liver – pleural effusions, ARDS, pulmonary calcification
Kidney – pulmonary oedema, pulmonary embolism, malignancy
Heart/lung – bronchiolitis obliterans

Cytomegalovirus pneumonia is a frequent and serious infection which prior to the advent of ganciclovir treatment proved fatal in transplant patients. Some units give human immunoglobulin prophylactically to protect against CMV in those patients who are CMV antibody negative. Prophylaxis against *Pneumocystis carinii* using septrin has been tried following transplantation. Inhaled pentamidine has not been studied in transplant patients as it has in AIDS but there is no theoretical reason why it should not be effective. Chest infection with fungi, especially aspergillus and candida, are frequent in transplant recipients. Studies have shown benefit from administering inhaled amphotericin B as prophylaxis against invasive aspergillosis in granulocytopenic patients after bone marrow transplantation.

In investigating pulmonary infection after transplant, sputum is generally regarded as inadequate or contaminated, and open lung biopsy has a significant morbidity. Bronchoalveolar lavage is established as useful in diagnosing opportunistic lung infections in transplant patients. The reduced platelet counts or deranged clotting time seen after some forms of transplantation can be a contraindication to transbronchial biopsy, but bronchoalveolar lavage itself is safe and does not cause bleeding complications. Transthoracic needle biopsies have been performed, but this procedure may be capable of disseminating aspergillosis through the bloodstream.

Conventionally, bacterial colony counts of less than 10^3/ml in lavage fluid are taken to suggest upper airway contamination, and counts of over 10^5/ml have been taken to mean pneumonia. Lavage can be a poor way of diagnosing aspergillus, as this organism tends to grow in vascular structures rather than in the alveolar lumen. In some centres 'surveillance' lavage is performed in bone marrow transplant recipients. If CMV is found one month after transplant, a 2-week course of ganciclovir can reduce the subsequent incidence of CMV pneumonia.

Non-infectious complications can depend on the type of transplant performed. The drugs and radiation used on patients prior to bone marrow transplantation can produce lung damage and the most frequent cause of death in the early period is DAH. Bronchiolitis obliterans can cause an obstructive lung disease and is relatively frequent in bone marrow transplant recipients and following lung transplantation. In both cases, it is a symptom of chronic rejection.

After liver transplantation, the commonest lung complication is a pleural effusion, usually a right sided transudate. This may be secondarily infected, and around 30% of cases will require a chest drain. Acute respiratory distress syndrome (ARDS) usually occurs within 2 weeks of liver transplant, and is usually secondary to another complication. Pulmonary calcification (usually asymptomatic) can occur in the first several months after liver transplant.

After kidney transplantation, pulmonary oedema can occur due to fluid overload and pulmonary embolism can be quite frequent. Later complications can be non-Hodgkin's lymphoma, Kaposi's sarcoma, and metastatic renal cell carcinoma.

After lung or heart–lung transplantation, rejection of lung is the most important complication. There is shortness of breath, fever, diffuse alveolar infiltrate and a rapidly progressive drop in pO_2. Bronchoscopy is essential to exclude any infection and transbronchial biopsy is usually performed to visualize the perivascular infiltration with lymphocytes. This is important, as the therapy involves increased immunosuppression which would make infection worse.

Prompt diagnosis of lung complications of transplantation is vital and both the infectious and non-infectious complications should be familiar to the infectious diseases specialist.

Further reading

ETTINGER, N. A. and TRULOCK, E. P. (1991) Pulmonary considerations of organ transplantation. *Am. Rev. Respir. Dis.*, **143**, 1386–1390.

Case 37   Needle-stick injury to a house officer

A house officer on a medical firm sustained a needle-stick injury having drawn blood by venipuncture. The source patient was suspected to be an intravenous drug-user and was admitted as an emergency with a diagnosis of endocarditis. The house officer immediately washed his hands, including the affected left index finger, with chlorhexidine and water and called his SHO for help.

Questions

1. What immediate information is required?
2. What action should be taken?

Answers

1. (i) Does the patient fall into a high risk category for transmission of hepatitis B virus (HBV), hepatitis C virus (HCV) or human immunodeficiency virus (HIV)?
   (ii) Was the needle (or sharp device) contaminated with the patient's blood?
   (iii) How deep was the injury?
   (iv) Did the house officer previously have a course of hepatitis B vaccination and is he known to be immune to this virus?
   (v) Is there a hospital policy for dealing with such 'sharps' injuries involving blood or body fluid exposure and where is it or who knows what it says?

   These questions are important for the risk assessment regarding the possible transmission of HBV, HCV or HIV to the house officer.

2. The following must be considered depending on the information acquired in 1.
   (i) If the house officer is HBV immune (anti-HBS antibody titre > 100 mIU/ml when tested within the last 2 years), no further action is generally needed regarding this virus. If the victim's immunity is waning, opportunity should be taken to administer a booster dose of vaccine.
   (ii) If the house officer was not immune to HBV, and risk assessment suggests possible transmission, then an accelerated course of HBV vaccination should be given as soon as possible and hepatitis B immunoglobulin should be administered if the source proves to be positive.
   (iii) A baseline sample of serum must be obtained from the house officer and stored to help document seroconversion to one of the viruses mentioned above.
   (iv) The hospital policy on zidovudine use in this setting should be applied. If the policy permits giving it, and the risk assessment suggests that HIV transmission is a possibility, then zidovudine should be given immediately (within 1–2 h of exposure).
   (v) There is no prophylactic regimen available for HCV and the house officer should be followed-up with liver function tests and serology.
   (vi) Depending on the risk assessment and actions taken, he should be referred for expert advice and counselling.
   (vii) An incident report must be filed according to hospital policy.

It is clear that if the exact status of the patient source is known then much distress can be avoided, but on-call virology services may not allow such rapid testing of samples for HIV, HBV and HCV. In practice, a number of the above-mentioned points occur simultaneously. The most successful overall approach in hospital practice utilizes a policy and a named person or persons for implementing the policy, such as the Occupational Health Physician by day and on-call microbiologist at night. The risk of transmission of HBV from a patient who is hepatitis B antigen positive following blood exposure in non-immune staff is about 30%. The risk of HIV transmission is less than 0.5%. The exact risk for HCV transmission is not fully determined, but is probably between 3 and 10%. Expert counselling is particularly important in explaining the risks and benefits of early zidovudine therapy.

Further reading

WORKING GROUP OF THE ROYAL COLLEGE OF PATHOLOGISTS (1992) HIV infection: Hazards of transmission to patients and healthcare workers during invasive procedures. The Royal College of Pathologists (UK).
HODD (1995) Time to hit HIV, early and hard (Editorial). *N. Engl. J. Med.*, **333**, 450–451.

Case 38   Rash and fever in a 1-year-old boy

A 1-year-old boy was admitted to the paediatric ward with a fever for 1 week. His growth and development were normal for his age, and he had received the usual childhood immunizations. His GP suspected a 'viral infection' or otitis media and prescribed amoxycillin, but the antibiotic did not reduce the fever and the child was admitted to hospital.

On examination his temperature was 37.7°C (after some paracetamol), BP 101/63, pulse 180/min, and the respiratory rate was 54/min. There was a faint red rash on the trunk, bilateral conjunctival injection and the lips were dry and cracked. The palms and soles were very red as was the mouth and tongue.

Blood tests showed Hb 12.2 g/dl, WBC 17.5×10^9/l (50% neutrophils), platelets 504×10^9/l. The ESR was 110 mm/h.

An ECG confirmed a sinus tachycardia with flattened T waves. Examination of the urine showed white cells but there was no subsequent bacterial growth. Antinuclear antibodies and rheumatoid factor were absent.

Questions

1. What is the next investigation?
2. What is the treatment?

Answers

1. Emergency echocardiography to search for aneurysmal dilatation of the coronary arteries.
2. Oral aspirin 80 mg/kg in four equal doses for 2 weeks, followed by a single daily dose of 4 mg/kg aspirin for a further 4 weeks. A single dose of intravenous immunoglobulin (1 g/kg) should also be given.

Comment

This is a typical history for Kawasaki syndrome, also known as the mucocutaneous lymph node syndrome. This presents with fever, rash and red conjunctivae suggestive of a viral infection, and this impression can be strengthened by the lack of response to antibiotics.

The syndrome was first described by Tomisaku Kawasaki in a Japanese medical journal in 1967. The illness usually affects children under 4, mostly boys and the disease usually strikes in the late winter or early spring. It often has a self-limiting course, but the main problem with missing the diagnosis is the possibility of cardiac complications.

The typical patient has a spiking fever, occasionally over 40°C, that continues without explanation for 5 or more days. Also, four of the five clinical criteria in Table 1 must be present, and these can be noted by a systematic head to toe examination.

Table 1: Clinical criteria for Kawasaki syndrome

EYES – Bilateral bulbar conjunctivitis without exudate
MOUTH – Redness in the oropharynx (often with dry cracked lips and red tongue)
NECK – Cervical lymphadenopathy (50–75% of patients)
HANDS/FEET – peripheral limb changes include oedema and/or redness in the palms and soles
TRUNK – A diffuse non-vesicular rash

As well as these diagnostic features, other findings can include joint pains, diarrhoea, ear pain, cough, dyspnoea, meningism, and elevation of hepatic transaminases.

The most dreaded complications are cardiac and these include myocarditis, coronary artery aneurysm, thrombosis, and myocardial infarction. In this case, the tachycardia out of proportion to the fever may have been a manifestation of myocarditis.

Laboratory tests usually show an elevated ESR, leucocytosis, thrombocytosis, moderate elevation of the AST and elevated CRP. The ANF and RhF are negative and ECG can show ST segment, T wave or QRS abnormalities.

The syndrome generally runs in three phases (Table 2).

Table 2: The three phases of Kawasaki syndrome, with approximate times

1.	Acute febrile phase (day 1–day 14)
2.	Subacute febrile phase (day 14–day 25)
3.	Convalescent phase (day 25–day 56)

In the first phase, all the clinical diagnostic findings are present, and very rarely the presentation can be with unilateral cervical lymphadenopathy and fever. In the subacute febrile stage, early signs resolve, and desquamation of the skin of the fingers and toes occurs, beginning in the nail areas. It is in the second phase that cardiac complications can be noted, but coronary artery aneurysms can actually appear on day 7 if looked for by echocardiography or MRI. In the convalescent phase, the signs and acute phase reactants return to normal.

Kawasaki syndrome is a vasculitis affecting small- and medium-sized arteries and affects the coronary arteries in particular. Coronary artery disease develops in 25% of those with untreated Kawasaki syndrome and this can lead to infarction and sudden death. In children under 7 months, peripheral ischaemia and gangrene can occur and this may need treatment with prostaglandin El with careful cardiac monitoring.

The treatment of Kawasaki syndrome aims to prevent cardiac complications and this can be achieved by the administration of high dose aspirin which prevents coronary artery thrombosis. Since 1986 it has been known that gamma globulin is effective in this syndrome, and that one dose of gamma globulin should be given early in the course of illness. A second echocardiogram at 6 weeks is often performed, and if this is normal, and the ESR is normal, the aspirin can be stopped. If an aneurysm is detected initially, but has resolved in 6 weeks then low dose aspirin is usually continued indefinitely. If an aneurysm is seen at 6 weeks then low dose aspirin is continued and yearly stress tests and perhaps angiography can be performed.

The cause of Kawasaki syndrome is unknown, but the selective expansion of V beta 2+T cells in the acute phase of the illness (both in peripheral blood and in the myocardium), suggests that the illness is triggered by a bacterial super-antigen, and indeed associations have been found between streptococcal infection and Kawasaki syndrome. Other suspected agents include Epstein-Barr virus and parvovirus.

Another recent development is the discovery of Kawasaki syndrome in adults infected with HIV, and although Kawasaki syndrome is occasionally described in adults, an HIV test should be considered in this situation.

Further reading

BELL, D. M., BRINK, E. W., NITZKIN, J. L. *et al.* (1981) Kawasaki syndrome: description of two outbreaks in the United States. *N. Engl. J. Med.*, **304**: 1568–1576.

Case 39   Acute pancreatitis as a biphasic illness

A 61-year-old man was on the waiting list for elective cholecystectomy for gallstones when he developed acute upper abdominal pain with a high serum amylase. The diagnosis of acute pancreatitis was made and he appeared to be making a good recovery with supportive measures. Two weeks after the onset of illness he again developed acute symptoms with abdominal pain, fever and leucoyctosis to $14 \times 10^9/l$.

Questions

1. What diagnosis must now be considered?
2. How may the diagnosis be confirmed?
3. What empirical antimicrobial regimen would you advise and why?

Answers

1. Superimposed infection of the pancreas must now be suspected; in some cases the pancreatic tissue may still be solid, whilst in others there may be a defined collection of pus (pancreatic abscess). Pancreatic abscess occurs in about 2–5% of patients following acute pancreatitis regardless of underlying cause (such as biliary stones, alcohol, or trauma).
2. The clinical features associated with infection of the pancreas are non-specific, although a relapse after initial recovery from the acute illness is highly suggestive. Abdominal pain and tenderness, nausea, vomiting and fever are frequent findings. CT scanning may show areas of regional necrosis and collections of pus. Many authorities suggest that percutaneous needle aspiration of pancreatic tissue and collections is safe under CT guidance and affords bacteriological culture for a clear separation of infected and non-infected cases.
3. For collections of pus, therapy must include surgical drainage and debridement as mortality is exceedingly high in patients with undrained collections. Antimicrobial therapy should cover the Enterobacteriaceae, *Enterococcus, Staphylococcus aureus* and anaerobic Gram-negative bacilli with broad spectrum agents or combinations, e.g. imipenem. It is noteworthy that though hypothetically useful, prophylactic antimicrobials in early pancreatitis do not appear to prevent subsequent development of abscess and may in fact promote drug resistance.

Further reading

D'Egidio, A. and Schein, M. (1991) Surgical strategies in the treatment of pancreatic necrosis and infection. *Br. J. Surg.*, **78**, 133–137.

Case 40   Fever, rash and possible sexual abuse

A 10-year-old girl was admitted to hospital with a 1-week history of malaise, fever and, in the few hours prior to admission, a skin rash and swelling of her right knee. The possible diagnosis of meningococcaemia had been raised by her family practitioner who had administered parenteral penicillin just prior to hospital referral. On admission, she was pyrexial with a temperature of 38.2°C but other vital signs were normal. There were no signs of meningeal irritation. There was a maculo-papular rash on the arms and legs with a few pustules. The right knee was swollen and tender. A light discharge was noted on her undergarments which closer examination revealed to be vaginal in origin. Attempted aspiration of the swollen right knee joint was unsuccessful but a Gram-stain performed on the miniscule amount of fluid exuded from the tip of the needle showed many polymorphs and a few Gram-negative diplococci. The CSF obtained by a lumbar puncture was normal for cells, glucose and protein and no organisms were seen. The child was on an 'at risk' register held by social services and the possibility of sexual abuse was mentioned to the registrar.

Questions

1. What are the two major diseases to consider?
2. What particular issues arise with specimen collection in suspected child abuse?
3. What are the implications for laboratory handling of such specimens?

Answers

1. Considering the history, physical signs, and the presence of Gram-negative diplococci on needle aspiration, the diagnosis is meningococcaemia or gonococcaemia. Meningococcaemia without meningitis can be even more fulminating than meningococcal meningitis and the child should be transferred to the Intensive Care Unit. The family practitioner acted appropriately by administering penicillin on first suspi-

cion of meningococcal illness. Strains of *N. meningitidis* continue to be penicillin sensitive in most of the world, including the United Kingdom. Strains of *N. gonorrhoeae* causing disseminated gonococcal infection (DGI) tend to be penicillin sensitive. However, if penicillin-resistant strains represent a significant proportion of isolates from urethritis and cervicitis, then bacteraemia from penicillin-resistant *N. gonorrhoeae* will also increase. Therefore, penicillin may or may not be appropriate empirical therapy for DGI. As the frequency of penicillin-resistant isolates increases, cefotaxime or ciprofloxacin may become more appropriate. Patients with DGI, though bacteraemic, may not show significant systemic illness. All cases of DGI arise from associated mucosal infection with *N. gonorrhoeae* but such infection may be asymptomatic. In this case, *N. gonorrhoeae* of the same serotype was isolated from a vaginal swab and blood cultures. Note that in the prepubertal girl, gonococcal infection of the lower genital tract is more of a vaginitis than a cervicitis.

2. Suspected child abuse is a clinical, psychosocial and medicolegal problem. The diagnosis of gonorrhoea in a child almost always indicates abuse and appropriate investigations are triggered by such diagnosis. It is vitally important that specimens for *N. gonorrhoeae* and other sexually transmissible pathogens are collected according to a locally agreed protocol by an experienced physician. Documentation on specimens and request forms must be thorough, since the resulting data may be required in legal proceedings. Results must only be sent to named agreed persons in order to maintain confidentiality.

3. In suspected child abuse, all laboratory protocols employed for *N. gonorrhoeae* and other sexually transmissible pathogens must ensure maximal sensitivity and specificity. Culture is still the 'gold standard' for diagnosis of gonorrhoea and is the method which is legally acceptable. Isolates should be kept indefinitely pending the need to send to reference laboratories or anywhere directed by a court-of-law.

Further reading

RAWSTON, S. A., BROMBERG, K. and HAMMERSCHLAG, M. R. (1993) STD in children: syphilis and gonorrhoea. *Genitourin. Med.*, **69**, 66–75.

DYSON, C. and HOSEIN, I. K. (1996) The role of the microbiology laboratory in the investigation of child sexual abuse. *J. Med. Microbiol.*, **45**, 1–6.

Case 41   A child with fever and diarrhoea

A 3-year-old boy was admitted to a paediatric ward because of fever and diarrhoea. He was developing normally except that his weight was below the 50th percentile. Two months before admission, he had been admitted to the hospital with cough, wheeze and fever and was given 7 days of oral amoxycillin and salbutamol by nebulizer. Two weeks before admission he again spent 7 days on the same ward receiving amoxycillin for cough and wheeze. Two days after discharge he developed diarrhoea with eight loose stools a day. He looked unwell, was feverish, had started vomiting and was therefore readmitted. His 5-year-old brother, who was also gaining weight along the 50th percentile, was well. Both parents were well and of normal height.

On examination the temperature was 37.2°C, BP 85 mmHg systolic and he appeared to be rather sleepy. Examination of the lungs demonstrated crackles at both bases. The heart and CNS were normal. The abdomen was distended with very few bowel sounds but the on-call surgeon found no evidence of an 'acute abdomen'.

Investigation showed HB 13.0 g/dl, WBC 31.2×10^9/l (57% neutrophils), ESR 3 mm/h, platelets 209×10^9/l, clotting screen normal, sodium 129 mmol/l, potassium 5.9 mmol/l, urea 10 mmol/l, creatinine 80 μmol/l, LFTs normal, albumin 14 g/l. Blood gases on air were PO_2 64 mmHg, PCO_2 30 mmHg, pH 7.4. Cerebrospinal fluid obtained by lumbar puncture showed clear fluid, two neutrophils and two lymphocytes/mm^2, glucose 3.0 mmol/l; no organisms were found on Gram-stain and antigen tests for *H. influenzae*, *S. pneumoniae* and *N. meningitidis* were negative.

Microscopy of stool showed moderate numbers of neutrophils; bacterial cultures for salmonella, shigella and campylobacter were negative. Electron microscopy for viral particles was also negative.

A chest X-ray was reported: 'Bilateral lower lobe infiltrates suggestive of pneumonia' and the abdominal X-ray was reported: 'Dilated loops of small bowel with air-fluid levels.' Cultures of blood, urine and CSF were negative, as was HIV serology.

Questions

1. What is the most likely cause of the diarrhoea?
2. What might predispose the child to this condition?

Answers

1. *Clostridium difficile.*
2. Multiple courses of antibiotics in hospital.

Comments

This child is very ill with a distended abdomen, hypoxia and severe diarrhoea that is producing dehydration. The white cell count is high, the albumin is low and neutrophils are seen in the stools.

Diarrhoea can be infectious or non-infectious in origin and non-infectious causes would include ulcerative colitis, Crohn's disease, coeliac disease and disaccharidase deficiency.

However, the onset of this illness appears to be acute and so infectious processes must be considered first. These may be divided into viral, bacterial and parasitic causes. Parasites, most commonly giardia and cryptosporidium, would not produce an inflammatory diarrhoea with neutrophils in the stool. Rotavirus can produce potentially fatal disease and is often seen in conjunction with respiratory illness; large numbers of viral particles are found in stool by electron microscopy. More commonly now an enzyme immunoassay for viral antigen is used. In this case, the high peripheral blood white cell count and the neutrophils in the stool suggest bacterial infection.

Responsible agents might include *E.coli* 0157: H7 which can not only produce bloody diarrhoea due to haemorrhagic colitis, but also the haemolytic uraemic syndrome or thrombocytopenic purpura and this agent should be excluded by specific culture. *Yersinia enterocolitica* can produce dysentery and pain mimicking acute appendicitis but is rare in the United Kingdom. Salmonella, shigella and campylobacter were not cultured in the stool. This is important because *Shigella* dysenteriae type I can produce septicaemia, dehydration, a leukaemoid reaction and air fluid levels on plain film of the abdomen, just as in this boy.

Because of the two recent hospital admissions involving administration of antibiotics, the most probable cause of this child's diarrhoeal illness is *Clostridium difficile*. Nosocomial infection with this organism is not uncommon and spores may be found throughout the hospital environment on floors, beds, and even telephones. Cross-infection is by the faecal–oral route. Alteration of the normal bowel flora by antibiotics such as ampicillin, cephalosporins or clindamycin allows *Clostridium difficile* to become established or overgrow in the large intestine. *C. difficile* secretes two exotoxins, A and B which damage the colonic epithelium. Clinical features can be of severe colitis with fever, dehydration, leucocytosis, diminished bowel sounds and a low albumin leading to peripheral oedema. Occasionally the diarrhoea may lessen though the patient's condition worsens from the combination of ileus and severe dehydration.

The recurrent chest infections and slow weight gain suggests another underlying disease especially as his brother is also small. Sweat test should be performed to exclude cystic fibrosis and immunoglobulins should be checked to look for IgA deficiency. An IgA deficient child may be prone to severe clostridial disease because of the failure to produce antibodies against the type A toxin.

The child should undergo sigmoidoscopy and biopsy for histology and stool examination for *C. difficile* toxin. Standard treatment for *C. difficile* associated diarrhoea is to stop all contributory antibiotics if possible and administer oral vancomycin or metronidazole. If the clinical status precludes oral treatment then intravenous metronidazole may be effective.

Further reading

BARTLETT, J. G. (1992) Antibiotic-associated diarrhoea. *Clin. Infect. Dis.*, **15**, 573–581.

Case 42   An elderly man with chronic lymphocytic leukaemia and pneumonia

A 75-year-old man was troubled by chills and malaise and was admitted to hospital for investigation. Three years previously he had been investigated for fatigue and found to have a white cell count of $20 \times 10^9/l$, with mainly mature appearing lymphocytes.

These were identified as B-lymphocytes and subsequent haematological opinion was that he had chronic lymphatic leukaemia in stage A, with involvement of cervical and axillary regions and no splenomegaly. Survival was expected to be 7 years and he was left untreated. Six months after diagnosis, routine blood counts showed thrombocytopenia and this was thought to be autoimmune in aetiology. He did not improve with steroids, and therefore underwent splenectomy. Thereafter, he remained on 10 mg prednisolone a day as maintenance. He had remained well until 2 days previously when chills and a productive cough started. He dismissed this as a 'bug' apparently doing the rounds of his sheltered housing complex, but was persuaded to be admitted by his general practitioner. He did not have pets and was not exposed to birds.

Examination showed a temperature of 39°C, pulse 120/min, BP 150/90 mmHg. Enlarged lymph nodes were found in the neck and left axilla and auscultation of the chest revealed crackles at both lung bases. The heart, abdomen and central nervous system were normal, as was urinalysis.

Laboratory investigations showed Hb 11.5 g/dl, WBC 21.0×10^9/l, (75% mature lymphocytes), platelets 200×10^9/l, ESR 100 mm/h, sodium 132 mmol/l, potassium 3.1 mmol/l, urea and creatine normal. Calcium, phosphate, liver function tests were normal apart from an AST of 50 IU. Chest X-ray showed numerous round nodules throughout both lungs, approximately 1 cm in diameter. Sputum examination showed few neutrophils, Gram-positive cocci, Gram-negative rods and filamentous Gram-positive rods. Blood gases showed pO_2 60 mmHg, pCO_2 27 mmHg, pH 7.55. Three days later there was still no clinical response to empirically administered erythromycin and augmentin; repeat chest X-ray showed new pulmonary modules and the appearance of bilateral effusions. Admission and subsequent blood cultures remained sterile.

Questions

1 What are the likely diagnoses?
2 What is the next investigation?

Answers

1. Nocardiosis or legionella.
2. Bronchoscopy with culture of bronchoalveolar lavage fluid.

Comment

This patient has a productive cough, fever and lung shadows on a background of haematological malignancy, and these features are suggestive of an infective pneumonia. The prognosis of community-acquired pneumonia is known to be worse in those over 65 years of age, those with underlying malignancies, and in those with vital sign abnormalities such as respiratory rate greater than 30/min or blood pressure less than 90 mmHg systolic. In most cases management of community acquired pneumonia revolves around assessing the severity of the patient's illness and giving empirical antimicrobial therapy rather than awaiting a specific microbial diagnosis which will not be made in at least 50% of cases. Diagnosis can be attempted in retrospect with viral and atypical serology. Gram-stain and culture of sputum have been repeatedly shown to be of little value in the management of most cases of pneumonia. It is not possible to tell the difference between atypical or typical pneumonias on the basis of history, blood test or chest X-ray and therefore treatment should consist of cover against *Streptococcus pneumoniae* (the commonest bacterial pathogen) and also atypicals, including legionella.

In this case, the patient is immunocompromised due to chronic lymphatic leukaemia (which is well known to produce hypogammaglobulinaemia), and also prednisolone. Patients with CLL are prone to infection with *Strep. pneumoniae*, *H. influenzae* and *S.aureus*, but infections with protozoa, fungi and TB are not more common, reflecting intact T cell functions. However, prednisolone can suppress T cell function and this should be borne in mind in this situation.

Table 1 gives the differential diagnosis of multiple nodules on the lung in this context.

Table 1: Causes of pulmonary nodules and fever in CLL

Lung disease from CLL.
Pneumonia (bacterial or viral)
Invasive pulmonary aspergillosis
Pulmonary mucomycosis
Pulmonary candidiasis
Cryptococcosis
Pneumocystis
Tuberculosis
Legionella
Nocardia

Direct invasion of the chest in chronic lymphatic leukaemia is usually manifested by reticular shadowing on the chest X-ray rather than nodules. Nodules on a chest X-ray are rare with *Strep. pneumoniae*, *H. influenzae* and *Staph. aureus* pneumonia and staphylococcal septicaemia was excluded by multiple blood cultures. Failure of response to broad-spectrum antibiotic treatment should also raise the suspicion that this is not a 'typical' bacterial infection. Varicella pneumonia is unlikely without the rash of chickenpox, and cytomegalovirus pneumonitis does not occur with this small degree of immunosuppression. *Candida albicans* was not grown from blood cultures, and cryptococcal antigen should be measured in the serum. Tuberculosis should be considered and acid-fast staining done. Mycobacteria can occasionally appear as weakly staining 'beaded' or filamentous Gram-positive rods on Gram-staining. In a person of this age, reactivation of quiescent disease would be expected to produce apical shadowing; and, moreover, there were no old apical scars on the chest X-ray. Miliary tuberculosis produces fine reticulonodular shadowing rather than large nodules and is manifested mainly by weight loss and anorexia rather than by cough.

Legionella should always be considered as a cause of community acquired pneumonia especially in the immunocompromised. Some variants of Legionella can certainly produce pulmonary nodules and some can stain positively with AFB. It is worth remembering that there are 22 species of Legionella, and ten serological variants of *Legionella pneumophila*. Urine tests for antigen should not be used as a screen, as these only detect sero group I of *Legionella pneumophila*. Attempts should be made to grow Legionella on buffered charcoal yeast extract agar, with antibotics added for selectivity. Chest X-ray usually shows unilateral shadowing which later involves both sides. However, non-specific poorly defined round shadows can occur, and one-third of cases are complicated by pleural effusions. Blood and sputum cultures are usually negative and the best method of diagnosis is culture of bronchoscopically obtained washings. Immunofluorescent staining of bronchial washings is not as sensitive as culture because the species causing the infection may not be represented by a corresponding diagnostic antibody. Of cases of pneumonia that proceed to the Intensive Care Unit, the main pathogen is *Strep. pneumoniae*, followed by legionella. Therefore, a patient who is deteriorating with pneumonia should have rifampicin added to the original empirical regimen, of say cefuroxime and erythromycin, in order to provide better cover against Legionella.

In this case, disease was caused by *Nocardia asteroides*, a weakly acid-fast staining Gram-positive higher bacterium with a filamentous appearance. It can complicate CLL, sometimes with a subacute clinical course. *Nocardia asteroides* is widely distributed in the environment, but very rarely seen in sputum and therefore should be considered pathogenic when found. Nocardia can spread from the lung to brain, producing the appearance of multiple abscesses on CT scanning, and can also produce skin nodules. Nocardia are difficult to find on sputum microscopy, and culture may also be negative because of low numbers of organisms. Staining and culture of BAL fluid is very productive.

This diagnosis must be considered in a patient with progressive pneumonia unresponsive to standard therapy, especially with a background of malignancy. The treatment is with co-trimoxazole for a prolonged course (6 months to 1 year); empyema or brain abscesses may require surgical drainage.

Further reading

FEIGIN, D.S. (1986) Nocardiosis of the lung; chest radiographic findings in 21 cases. *Thorac. Radiol.*, **159**, 9–14.

HENKLE, J. Q. and NAIR, S. V. (1986) Endobronchial pulmonary nocardiosis. *JAMA*, **256**, 1331–1332.

Case 43   Ruptured aortic aneurysm

A 70-year-old male patient with a history of rheumatoid arthritis underwent transurethral resection of the prostate for benign prostatic hyperplasia. His urine had shown a significant growth of *E. coli*, and appropriate antibiotic cover with gentamicin was used at surgery. He made an unremarkable recovery until the fourth post-operative day when he become febrile to 38.4°C. Two days before this, a patient on the same four-bedded ward was noted to have had diarrhoea and bacterial culture of stool apparently yielded a significant isolate. The current patient did not have diarrhoea but continued to spike a temperature and sweat profusely over the next few days. Three sets of blood cultures were drawn over several hours and empirical therapy was started with intravenous cefotaxime. His urine was negative after culture but all blood cultures subsequently grew the same isolate as was found in the patient with diarrhoea. Infection in the case patient was attributed to cross-infection from the patient who developed diarrhoea. The invasiveness in the case patient was thought to have arisen because of his age and chronic steroid use for rheumatoid arthritis. He appeared to be making a favourable response when on the eighth post-operative day he died suddenly. At autopsy, the peritoneal cavity was completely filled with blood and a ruptured abdominal aortic aneurysm was noted. This aneurysm had been undetected prior to death.

Questions

1. To what genus is the organism likely to belong?
2. What are the usual laboratory tests employed for typing of isolates?
3. What was the clue that the organism had probably seeded an intravascular lesion?
4. What is the optimal management of such seeded intravascular foci?

Answers

1. The suggestion of cross-infection by an organism causing diarrhoea in one patient and bacteraemia with probable seeding of an abdominal aortic aneurysm in the other is highly suggestive of *Salmonella* sp.
2. Salmonella can be typed in most clinical laboratories by sero-agglutination and biochemical profiles (API 20E). This isolate was *Salmonella typhimurium*.
3. Transient bacteraemia with highly invasive serotypes such as *S. typhimurium* can occur as part of a gastrointestinal infection, particularly if there are predisposing factors such as age and chronic steroid use. On the other hand, Salmonellae have a unique predilection to seed sites of pre-existing structural damage such as bone and joints and, particularly in the cardiovascular system. A patient with a persistent bacteraemia strongly suggests a focal intracardiac or intravascular lesion. Cardiac sites include ventricular aneurysms and

damaged mural (as opposed to valvular) endocardium. Non-cardiac intravascular sites include atheromatous plaques and aneurysms of the abdominal aorta and ileo-femoral vessels.

4. If persistent bacteraemia is present, a search must be made for a cardiovascular site of infection by echocardiography and angiography. If a site is found then surgery must be considered as a priority because of the likely poor outcome with medical therapy only. Antimicrobial treatment is for 4–6 weeks as for endocarditis.

Further reading

COHEN, J. I., BARTLETT, J. A. and COREY, G. R. (1987) Extra-intestinal manifestations of salmonella infections. *Medicine*, **66**, 349–388.

Case 44   An HIV positive man with chronic diarrhoea

A 30-year-old homosexual arts theatre administrator arrived for a routine outpatient clinic, 6 weeks after having been in the hospital for investigation of chronic large volume diarrhoea.

Five years previously he had requested a routine HIV test at a genitourinary clinic and this was found to be positive. Three years previously he had developed chronic diarrhoea and 6 months prior to his recent hospital admission he had been noticed to have cytomegalovirus (CMV) retinitis and CMV colitis. These were treated using ganciclovir through a central line and granulocyte colony-stimulating factor was also needed for resulting neutropenia.

He was also taking fluconazole for oral candidiasis, monthly inhaled pentamidine for pneumocystis prophylaxis and zidovudine (AZT). Three weeks prior to the admission to hospital, he developed a cough productive of green sputum and fever. At that time he also noticed an increase in his diarrhoea to six large volume stools a day without presence of blood or mucus.

Perusing the notes of the hospital admission you see that he was found to be very thin with two lesions of Kaposi's sarcoma in the left lower leg. There was no lymphadenopathy, and examination of the left fundus showed scarring but no active CMV retinitis. His indwelling subclavian catheter appeared un-infected and neurological examination was normal. The lungs were clear, respiratory rate 16 per minute and the chest was normal with blood pressure 110/70. Blood result had shown Hb 10.1 g/dl, MCV 101 fl, WBC 1.6 (41% neutrophils), platelets $120 \times 10^9/l$. Urea, electrolytes and liver function tests were normal including albumin and globulin levels. A chest X-ray and abdominal X-ray were normal, blood cultures from veins and from central line showed no growth and staining of the sputum for *Pneumocystis carinii* was negative. However, there was a heavy growth of *H. influenzae* in the sputum. An MSU was clear.

A telephone call from the clinic to the microbiology laboratory establishes that blood and stool cultures for mycobacteria have been negative for the past 6 weeks.

Whilst in the hospital, he had been given cefuroxime i.v. and the cough and fever had settled. His diarrhoea also settled to three watery stools per day, which was normal for him. Examination of the stools for bacterial growth, parasites *Clostridium difficile* toxin and acid fast-bacilli had been negative. Looking through his notes you find a note that, smear of formalin-fixed stool stained with modified trichrome shows numerous pink oval bodies 2 microns in diameter.

Question

1. What is the diagnosis?
2. What further investigations would you perform?

Answers

1. Intestinal microsporidiosis.
2. Examination of a distal duodenal biopsy by electron microscopy.

Comment

Microsporidiosis is a well recognized cause of diarrhoea in patients with AIDS. It was found in 1992 that microsporidial spores could be identified with high specificity and sensitivity in stool using the modified trichrome stain and light microscopy, but being only 2 microns across they can be easily missed. Staining of duodenal biopsies with haematoxylin and eosin or Giemsa will show eosinophilic structures in the cytoplasm of enterocytes, especially in the villi and there may be no inflammation or villous blunting. Electron microscopy of enterocytes shows numerous 2 micron spores, between five and 25 contained in vacuoles. Detailed examination of the ultrastructure of spores will allow classification of the species. This classification can be important because although the commonest enteric microsporidium, *Enterocytozoon bienusi* is relatively resistant to treatment, another species *Septata intestinalis* may have a good response to albendazole. In microsporidiosis, albendazole is given for 3 months and a response is usually seen within a few weeks with weight gain and sometimes complete cessation of diarrhoea.

Metronidazole has also been evaluated for microsporidiosis, but symptoms can also relapse and remit spontaneously. As is typical of the small bowel pathogens, microsporidiosis does not produce fever, and the temperature in this case was caused by acute bronchitis due to *H. influenzae*, which was cleared by cefuroxime.

The typical patient with microsporidiosis passes six loose stools a day and has a CD4 count of less than $100/mm^3$. An interesting feature of microsporidiosis is a normal albumin in spite of diarrhoea and considerable weight loss.

Diarrhoea in AIDS has a small bowel-like or large bowel-like presentation. Small bowel pathogens produce large volume diarrhoea and occasionally malabsorption, whereas large bowel pathogens produce left-sided abdominal pain, small volume stools, blood and mucus. Routine investigation should include culture for salmonella, campylobacter and other bacteria, AFB staining for mycobacterium avium and cryptosporidium, stool examination for Giardia, *Isospora belli* and other parasites, and measurement of *Clostridium difficile* toxin. CMV colitis should be diagnosed by sigmoidoscopy and biopsy, as the evidence that CMV is the cause of a disease depends on demonstrating intranuclear inclusions in a biopsy specimen. Often the cause of diarrhoea cannot be found, and this is often attributed to direct infection of enterocytes by the HIV virus. Patients with high volume diarrhoea should be assessed for malabsorption using the xylose tolerance test, and measurement of vitamin B_{12}, folic acid and fat soluble vitamins in the blood. This is important in patients taking AZT who have a macrocytosis that may disguise the onset of B_{12} deficiency.

Pernicious anaemia is common in HIV infection even without small intestinal pathology, presumably due to infection of gastric parietal cells with HIV.

If no cause for diarrhoea can be found by stool examination then endoscopy and small bowel biopsy should be performed to look for intestinal parasites and mycobacteria.

Further reading

SHADDUCK, J. A. (1989) Human microsporidiosis and AIDS. *Rev. Infect. Dis.*, **11**, 203–207.

Case 45 A young woman on a renal ward with enterococcal bacteraemia

A 25-year-old woman with chronic renal failure on haemo-dialysis developed bacteraemia with a presumptively identified enterococcus resistant to vancomycin, teicoplanin and ampicillin. This was the second patient to develop an infection with this organism on the relevant renal ward. The ward was also known to have had an endemic problem with methicillin resistant *Staphylococcus aureus* (MRSA).

Questions

1. What are the options for antimicrobial therapy of the bacterae-mia?
2. What is the prognosis?
3. What is the potential for further spread of the vancomycin-resistant enterococcus (VRE)?

Answers

1. The number of reports of VRE continue to rise in the UK with *Enterococcus faecium* predominating. The best choice for empirical therapy of multiresistant strains is unknown with various regimens of chloramphenicol, quinolones, fucidin and aminoglycosides having been tried depending on specific

resistance patterns. Newer streptogramin compounds may have a role with *E. faecium* and are under investigation.

2. The prognosis with VRE bacteraemia is very much the same as with sensitive enterococci and reflects the severity of underlying disease. In the absence of optimal antimicrobial treatment, attention to potential sources of infection such as vascular lines or intra-abdominal collections assume vital importance and may decide the outcome.

3. The epidemiology of VRE is currently under intense investigation. A reasonable working approach is to consider VRE spread along similar lines to MRSA. In this regard, the organism is likely to spread if <u>hygiene fails</u> and <u>antimicrobial pressure</u> is sustained. It is noteworthy that the ward in question had an endemic MRSA problem so that we can expect vancomycin use to have been even greater than is usual for renal wards. It would be critical for the ward in question to review all antimicrobial policies and particularly those relating to glycopeptide use.

Comment

E. faecium resistant to penicillin and vancomycin was first reported in 1988 and world wide increases have been noted subsequently. In the UK, most isolates have been of the Van A phenotype (resistant to vancomycin and teicoplanin). The Van B phenotype (resistant to vancomycin but sensitive to teicoplanin) accounts for approximately 20% of clinically significant isolates. Most clusters have been in the renal, haematology and intensive care settings. Epidemiologic studies to date have suggested that spread of resistance can occur within strains (e.g. in the same patient) and between patients. The threat of VRE is that it will follow a similar epidemiologic curve to MRSA under selective antimicrobial pressures and contact spread. There is also the ever present danger of spread of glycopeptide resistance genes from VRE to MRSA, particularly since both frequently occur in the same patient population.

Further reading

EDMOND, M. B., OBER, J. F., WEINBAUM, D. L. *et al.* (1995) Vancomycin-resistant *Enterococcus faecium* bacteraemia: risk factors for infection. *Clinical Infectious Diseases*, **20**, 1126–1133.

Norris, A. H., Reilly, J. P., Edelstein, P. H. *et al.* (1995) Chloramphenicol for the treatment of vancomycin-resistant enterococcal infections. *Clinical Infectious Diseases*, **20**, 1137–1144.

Leclercq, R., Derlot, E., Duval, J. *et al.* (1988) Plasmid mediated resistance to vancomycin and teicoplanin in *Enterococcus faecium. N. Engl. J. Med.*, **319**, 157–161.

Case 46 — A boy with a swollen ankle and delirium

A 16-year-old boy scout suffered an insect bite above the left ankle while on a camping expedition. Within hours the area became hot, red and tender with a diffuse erythema involving the lower one-third of the leg. He was taken to a local family practitioner who prescribed an antihistamine ointment to be applied topically and oral penicillin 250 mg 4 times a day. During that night, the swelling and pain continued to increase and the erythema now extended over the entire leg below the knee. By next morning he was sweating profusely and in a delirious state and was admitted to hospital. Blood cultures were immediately drawn and intravenous antibiotic therapy commenced.

Questions

1. What is the likely diagnosis?
2. Was the pre-hospital management appropriate?
3. How is the condition distinguished from necrotizing fasciitis.

Answers

1. The likely diagnosis is Streptococcal cellulitis following introduction of the Group A streptococcus (*S. pyogenes*) on the skin surface into the deep dermis/subcutaneous fat by the insect bite. The diagnosis is essentially clinical, since in the vast majority of cases there is no primary open lesion and superficial skin swabs are negative. In the normal host, as in this case, the primary lesion may be a skin crack or minute puncture wound.
2. The initial management included penicillin in low dose but cellulitis can be a rapidly progressive disease that can lead

to bacteraemia, and treatment should be with parenteral antibiotics directed particularly against the Group A streptococcus. If the disease is regarded as being in the very initial
stages, then oral therapy may be effective provided that this
is with an agent in sufficient dosage likely to give adequate
blood levels, for example amoxycillin 500 mg tds. If the
patient is admitted to hospital, intravenous therapy is
always warranted. Although cellulitis of this nature following
insect bite in the normal host is most commonly caused
by the Group A streptococcus, *Staphylococcus aureus* has
occasionally been implicated as a co-pathogen and hence
staphylococcal cover should also be considered, with, say,
co-amoxiclav (augmentin) or flucloxacillin. These latter antimicrobials cover both Group A streptococcus and *S. aureus.*

3. This condition is a superficial spreading cellulitis which is
principally subcutaneous and does not involve the muscle
layer in the region affected – a major finding in necrotizing
fasciitis. Clinically, the distinction can be difficult, but most
cases of infection following these minor traumatic problems
such as insect bite tend to be of the superficial cellulitic type.
Having said this, the presence of extensive ecchymosis, bulla
formation, cutaneous gangrene, anaesthesia, or failure to improve on appropriate parenteral antibotics should prompt a
surgical consultation for possible exploration. In necrotizing
fasciitis blunt dissection following skin incision shows disin-
tegration of the fascial plane with extensive undermining.

Comment

The American literature in particular suggests that more severe
group A streptococcal infections are now being seen, including
those associated with a toxic-shock-like syndrome. In addition,
increases in acute rheumatic fever have also been reported.

Further reading

BRYAN, B. O. and FRIEDEN, I. (1992) Streptococcal skin disease in children. *Semin.
Dermatol.*, **11**, 3–10.
STEVENS, D. L., TANNER, H. M., WINSHIP, J. *et al* (1989) Severe group A streptococcal
infections associated with toxic shock-like syndrome and scarlet fever toxin
A. *N. Engl. J. Med.*, **321**, 1–7.

Case 47   An Ecuadorian student with a seizure

A 25-year-old man from Ecuador was an exchange student in the United Kingdom for a period of 2 years. He was admitted to hospital with an acute severe headache unresponsive to paracetamol and a suspected diagnosis of bacterial or viral meningitis. He had been generally well but recalled a family member in Ecuador having had some form of bowel infection. Soon after admission he developed a focal seizure. A CT scan showed cystic lesions 0.5 to 1.0 cm in diameter scattered throughout the cerebral parenchyma, some of which had calcified.

Questions

1. Considering all the evidence presented what is the likely diagnosis?
2. What are the various modes of presentation?
3. What is the treatment?

Answers

1. The most likely diagnosis is neurocystcercosis caused by *Taenia solium*; world-wide, this is the most common parasitosis affecting the nervous system. Salient points to note in the history are:
   (i) Origin from an endemic region – the disease is common in Latin America, Asia, Africa and some parts of Eastern Europe;
   (ii) History of a possible parasitosis in a family member;
   (iii) The presentation with acute headache which frequently arises from acute, life threatening hydrocephalus. In this case the headache occurred due to meningeal involvement;
   (v) The CT scan appearance is virtually diagnostic;

2. It should be recalled that cysticercosis arises from the migration of the larvae of *T. solium* in the human host – a phase which should occur in the intermediate host, the pig. The larvae are transported by blood and lymphatic vessels from the intestinal wall and lodge particularly in brain, skeletal muscle and

subcutaneous tissues. In the CNS clinical features depend on the location of cysts and the host inflammatory response. The patient may be asymptomatic with cysts or present with epilepsy, acute hydrocephalus or meningoencephalitis. With meningeal involvement CSF frequently shows a lymphocytic pleocytosis and elevated protein. Eosinophilia is not an uncommon finding in peripheral blood and CSF. Serological tests for specific antibody are frequently positive (ELISA, indirect haemagglutination).

3. The drug of choice which kills viable larvae is praziquantel and patients without hydrocephalus can be expected to respond very well. An exacerbation of symptoms from a strong inflammatory reaction in the first few days of treatment can be suppressed with steroids. Praziquantel has also been used in large scale 'epidemiologic' treatment of populations in endemic areas to decrease the reservoir of *T. solium.*

Further reading

CRUZ, M., CRUZ, I. and HORTON, J. (1991) Albendazole versus praziquantel in the treatment of cerebral cystercercosis. *Trans. R. Soc. Trop. Med. Hyg.*, **85**, 244–247.

Case 48　A child with hepatosplenomegaly and lymphocytosis

A 3-year-old boy with no particular problems was taken by his mother to see the general practitioner because of a runny nose and cough. He was prescribed amoxicillin, but after 2 days a petechial rash appeared and re-examination by the general practitioner showed that the liver and spleen were now palpable. He was admitted to hospital.

He was born at term with a normal delivery and normal birth weight. He had received all the usual immunizations, and there were no family pets. He had not been abroad and his sister of 5 years old and parents were well.

On examination he appeared listless, was apyrexial with blood pressure of 100/40 and pulse 100/min. There was a petechial rash over the trunk, arms and legs and shotty lymph nodes could be felt in the neck, axillae, and groins. There was no headache, meningism or photophobia, and auscultation of the heart and lungs was normal. A liver edge could be palpated 4 cm below the costal margin and the spleen was felt 6cm below the left costal margin.

Investigation showed Hb 10.4 g/dl, WBC 17.4 × 10^9/l (40% lymphocytes, atypical cells seen) platelets 12 × 10^9/l clotting screen normal, sodium 138 mmol/l, potassium 4.4 mmol/l, urea and creatinine normal. Calcium and phosphate levels were normal and a monospot test was negative.

Questions

1. What are the two most likely diagnoses?
2. What further investigation should be considered with this clinical picture?

Answers

1. Infection with Epstein–Barr virus or cytomegalovirus.
2. Examination of a bone marrow to exclude acute leukaemia.

Comment

This child presents with hepatosplenomegaly, atypical lymphocytosis, thrombocytopenia and a petechial rash. A petechial rash can result from damage to blood vessel walls, or from low levels of poor functioning of platelets. A platelet count of 12 × 10^9/l would account for the petechiae in this case. Low platelet counts can be caused by decreased production from the bone marrow, for example following infiltration in acute leukaemia or histiocytosis, and therefore the atypical cells should be examined further. Thrombocytopenia can also follow increased platelet destruction produced by conditions such as immune thrombocytopenia, either idiopathic or following specific infectious disease. Haemolytic uraemic syndrome and thrombotic thrombocytopenic purpura are unlikely in this case, as no microangiopathic haemolytic picture was seen on blood films, and there is no renal impairment. Disseminated intravascular coagulation is only very rarely seen in these two conditions, and they cannot be excluded by the normal clotting screen.

Idiopathic immune thrombocytopenia commonly affects small children but does not produce lymphadenopthy or hepatosplenomegaly. Also, the blood film is usually normal apart from thrombocytopenia and no atypical cells are seen. Thrombocytopenia can follow specific viral infection such as Epstein–Barr virus, cytomegalovirus, or may follow brucellosis or cat scratch disease. These last two are unlikely without a specific history of appropriate exposure.

Although histiocytosis can give rise to lymphadenopathy or hepatosplenomegaly, again atypical lymphocytes are not a feature, and he is rather old for a first presentation of this disease. The possibility of a metabolic storage disease producing hepatosplenemegaly and lymphadenopathy is very unlikely as the child would have suffered some developmental delay and failure to thrive.

Examination of the blood film showed a heterogeneous appearance of the atypical cells, making acute leukaemia unlikely. However, bone marrow biopsy might still be performed to exclude infiltration of the marrow.

Infective causes of atypical lymphocytosis are Epstein–Barr virus, cytomegalovirus, infectious hepatitis, toxoplasmosis, syphilis, brucellosis and various other viruses. Whooping cough can also produce this picture but vaccination for this disease had been given already. By far the most likely causes are cytomegalovirus and Epstein–Barr virus.

Cytomegalovirus infection in childhood is usually asymptomatic, but is often accompanied by lymphocytosis and mild elevation in levels of aspartate transaminase and alkaline phosphatase. Thrombocytopenia can complicate CMV in around one in 30 cases, and as well as serology, urine culture could be attempted.

Epstein–Barr virus infects B cells and the lymphocytosis in the blood is caused by an increase in CD8+ T cells that are controlling the viral infection. The B cells themselves are mainly in the lymph nodes, rather than circulating in the blood. Epstein–Barr virus infection is very common in childhood and is usually not clinically apparent. However, children under 4 years are more likely to develop symptoms, and there is a high rate of splenomegaly, hepatomegaly and respiratory tract symptoms as in this case. Other manifestations are a failure to thrive and oedema of the eyelids. In childhood, EBV infection is almost always accompanied by lymphocytosis but the monospot and Paul Bunnell tests are usually negative, as in this instance. In 90% of cases there is an elevated AST, and the bilirubin is raised in around half the cases. Thrombocytopenia is unusual and hardly ever serious and steroids or immune globulin can be used for treatment. The mechanism of thrombocytopenia involves the development of antiplatelet antibodies. Epstein–Barr virus can also produce a haemophagocytic syndrome, which would be manifested by a pancytopenia and abnormalities of coagulation.

A bone marrow biopsy will reveal differences between EBV infection and leukaemia by showing a normocellular bone marrow in EBV infection with perhaps increased numbers of megakaryocytes and a lymphocytosis. Flow cytometery studies will show that 80% of the T cells are CD8 positive, CD2 positive, CD5 positive and HLADR positive.

In this case confirmation of EBV infection would be obtained by measuring IgM and IgG antiviral antibodies.

Further reading

Tosato, G. and Blaese, R. M. (1985) Epstein–Barr virus infection and immunoregulation in man. *Adv. Immunol.*, **27**: 99.

Case 49   Post-gastroenteritis paraesthesia

A 23-year-old male student developed severe abdominal pain and diarrhoea and was admitted to hospital with a possible diagnosis of acute appendicitis or enteric infection. He ate out quite frequently and had had *Salmonella* gastroenteritis 6 months previously. On examination, he was distressed with apparent rebound tenderness in the lower abdomen; vital signs were: pulse 92/min, respiratory rate 24/min, blood pressure 130/70 mmHg and temperature 38.1°C. Emergency laparotomy was performed and the appendix, though not inflamed looking, was removed. Three days later the histopathologist reported a normal appendix and the microbiology laboratory then reported a stool culture positive for *Campylobacter jejuni.* He made an uneventful recovery with supportive measures only and was discharged home on the fifth post-operative day. Two weeks later he noticed 'pins and needles' in his feet which then progressed to muscle weakness of the legs and arms and the complaint of 'becoming tired breathing'. He was readmitted for investigation.

Questions

1. What is the likely clinical diagnosis?
2. What is the CSF likely to show?
3. What is the prognosis?
4. What is the therapy?

Answers

1. Guillain–Barré syndrome (GBS) following *Campylobacter* enteric infection. Campylobacteriosis is a recognized predisposing infection along with influenza, cytomegalovirus and *Mycoplasma pneumoniae* amongst others. The syndrome usually begins 1–4 weeks after an acute respiratory or gastro-intestinal infection or immunization with progressive paraesthesiae and symmetric limb weakness. *Campylobacter jejuni* is emerging as the most common preceding infection and particular strains may be involved. On examination there is a flaccid paralysis and loss of deep tendon reflexes. The Miller–Fisher variant of Guillain–Barré may resemble botulism but a prominent ataxia in the former is lacking in the latter.
2. Lumbar puncture performed early in the disease may be normal but protein becomes elevated later. The CSF white cell count is usually less than 20 lymphocytes/ml.
3. Most patients recover over weeks to months but fatalities can occur due to complications: such as respiratory failure, cardiac arrythmias and pulmonary embolism. Chronic variants of the disease have been described.
4. Plasmapheresis is standard therapy in acute GBS and in the chronic variant, chronic inflammatory demyelinating radiculoneuropathy, and is performed about 5 times over 1–2 weeks. Intravenous immunoglobulin has also been used.

Further reading

ROPPER, A. H. (1988) Campylobacter diarrhoea and Guillain-Barré syndrome. *ARCL Neurol*, **45**, 655.

Case 50 A young woman with a history of a fractured right femoral shaft and chronic discharging sinuses

You are consulted about a 35-year-old female who suffered a mid-shaft fracture of the right femur in a road traffic accident. She made an uneventful recovery following internal fixation with an intramedullary nail. One year later, the nail was removed because of recurrent discharging sinuses and episodes of pain suggestive of chronic osteomyelitis unresponsive to antimicrobial therapy. She continued to have discharging sinuses and bone and gallium scans suggested residual osteomyelitis. One year post-removal of the nail she is still on oral flucloxacillin even though no organism was ever grown from deep bone removed and submitted for culture at the time of nail removal. Superficial wound swabs have grown *Proteus* species and *S. aureus* on a number of occasions. She is pain free, apyrexial and has a normal peripheral blood white cell count.

Question

1. Will you continue with the flucloxacillin?

Answer

1. All forms of acute osteomyelitis may progress to chronic disease with varying degrees of bone loss, persistent drainage and sinus tracts. The cornerstone of management is the removal of foci of infected bone together with antimicrobial therapy. The isolation of causative organisms in chronic osteomyelitis is vital not just to establish the diagnosis, but also to allow for antimicrobial sensitivity testing and selection of specific antibiotics. In this case, the information given strongly suggests chronic bone infection at the time the nail was removed, even though no organism was grown. 'No growth' does not mean 'no microbial pathogens present', since failure to grow an organism may arise if the patient was on concurrent antibiotics to which such organism was susceptible. We must also make the assumptions that:

(i) The bone was not wrongly placed in formalin (and then removed when the mistake was realized in theatre).
(ii) The bone was transported to the laboratory quickly.
(iii) Patient demographics and specimen labelling were correct.
(iv) Laboratory processing was timely and used appropriate methods subject to necessary quality control systems.

Comment

These are all possible reasons, which are not infrequent by any means, for a mis-match between laboratory data and clinical suspicion. The superficial swab results may also encourage over reliance on a positive laboratory result. It is highly likely that any moist cutaneous lesion will become colonized with nearby 'normal flora'. In this patient, the perineum may have already been colonized with *S. aureus* and long-term antimicrobial therapy directed against Gram-positives would promote the growth of *Proteus* sp. (and other Gram-negatives).

We are therefore faced with the following:

(i) a clinical picture suggestive of chronic osteomyelitis;
(ii) radiological evidence of chronic infection;
(iii) the normal WBC and lack of fever are not unusual in chronic osteomyelitis;
(iv) no organism from deep bone cultures 1 year previously;
(v) superficial wound swab culture results which may not reflect what is deep;
(vi) patient on long-term flucloxacillin;

The logical plan would be to stop the flucloxacillin, and explore and debride the tracts and bone with submission of multiple samples for cultures. Antimicrobial therapy must not just be to 'cover' but be optimal considering all variables including infecting organism and pharmacokinetics. For example, if *S. aureus* was the target organism, the addition of fucidic acid or rifampicin to flucloxacillin (or vancomycin/teicoplanin for MRSA) may be decisive because of excellent tissue penetration.

Further reading

ANTHONY, J. P. and MATHES, S. J. (1991) Update on chronic osteomyelitis. *Clin. Plast. Surg.*, **18**: 515–523.

Case 51   Myalgia and acute renal failure

A 57-year-old warehouseman had been feeling out of sorts with painful muscles for 10 days before going to see his general practitioner. He was usually healthy and managed his job with no problems. The start of his illness had been marked by a headache which was throbbing over the forehead, diarrhoea and fever of 39°C. His general practitioner had seen him on the morning of admission to hospital, and sent blood samples which revealed that the creatinine was raised, and he was therefore admitted to the renal ward. He lived with his wife and two children in a suburban area and owned two dogs and a cat. There was no history of foreign travel or exposure to farm animals.

On examination he was alert but somewhat disorientated in time. His temperature was 39.8°C, BP 120/70 mmHg, pulse 100/min. There was no postural drop in the blood pressure. The conjunctivae were very hyperaemic. Examination of the chest was normal, but abdominal examination revealed slight distention and tenderness without rebound. Examination of the central nervous system was normal, and there was no neck stiffness.

Blood results were Hb 13.4 g/dl, WBC 10.4×10^9/l (94% neutrophils), platelets 70×10^9/l, sodium 123 mmol/l, potassium 3.8 mmol/l, urea 28.0 mmol/l, creatinine 500 μmol/l, bilirubin 241 μmol/l, gamma GT 70 IU/l, AST 70 IU/l. The alkaline phosphatase was normal. The creatine kinase was 1100 IU/l. The ESR was 114 mm/h, and a coagulation screen was normal.

Analysis of urine showed eight WBC and ten RBC per high power field without casts. Chest X-ray, abdominal X-ray and abdominal ultrasound were normal and blood and urine cultures were sterile.

Questions

1. What is the likely diagnosis?
2. What is the likely source of the problem?

Answers

1. Leptospirosis.
2. The family dogs.

Comment

Leptospira were not cultured from the blood in this case but they can be found during the first 10 days of illness using cultures on suitable media such as Tween-80-albumin.

These should have been incubated for 5–6 weeks at 28–30°C in darkness. As leptospira are viable in anticoagulated blood for up to 11 days, specimens can be sent for culture to a reference laboratory in a suggestive case but beware that citrate as an anticoagulant will kill leptospira. Antibodies to leptospira appear on day 6–12 of illness and reach a maximum titre in around 25 days. If antibiotics have been given, the rise in antibody may well be delayed and further tests should be performed at later periods to confirm the diagnosis. The serotype of the organism can only be determined if they are grown in culture, and this will prove to be important in establishing the source of infection.

Leptospira are spirochaetes that produce an extensive generalized vasculitis and humans are infected mainly through contact with animals. There is only one species pathogenic for humans, *Leptospira interrogans*, with more than 200 known serotypes. After penetrating mucous membranes or a cut in the skin, leptospira disseminate widely and can enter the cerebrospinal fluid and the eye. There is hepatic dysfunction that produces jaundice, and tubular damage resulting in renal failure. Renal impairment can also be produced by the low blood volume resulting from leakage of fluid through damaged endothelial cells. Myalgia can be very prominent, affecting 80% of patients, but histologically the findings in muscles are very mild. Leptospirosis is often accompanied by a meningitis, but this does not occur when leptospira are in the CSF during the first week, but rather after the appearance of antibodies and the disappearance of the organisms which suggest that this is an immune mediated effect.

Subclinical cases of leptospirosis are common. For example, 15% of veterinarians in the United States have evidence of previous exposure. Only 10% of patients affected with leptospirosis develop jaundice and renal impairment (Weil's disease) but the mortality of this condition is considerable up to 5–10%. The AST level in Weil's disease is very rarely high, and the finding of a relatively low level of transaminases in a very jaundiced patient should alert the physician to the diagnosis. Once jaundice has occurred, patients are at risk of renal failure and hypotension and although patients can develop thrombocytopenia, disseminated intravascular coagulation is rare.

If the patient is seen during the second week of illness when the blood and cerebrospinal fluid are free of leptospira, then isolation should be attempted from the urine which contains leptospira, from the second week onwards.

Dogs can be infected with *Leptospira interrogans serovar canicola*, and if there are family pets urine should be obtained from them by a veterinary surgeon and blood samples taken for leptospira antibody titres. There is still a risk that other family members could be affected, and up to 30% of human cases of leptospirosis are caused by contact with dogs.

Although it had been previously thought that antibiotic therapy is not effective after the first 4 days of illness, recent studies have indicated that antibiotics may in fact be effective at a late stage. Ampicillin, cefotaxime and doxycycline can save hamsters from experimentally-produced leptospirosis even late in the illness, and it is known that in humans penicillin G started even after day 5 can reduce the time spent in hospital and the elevation of creatinine. Therefore, in severely ill patients (such as this case) treatment with either penicillin G or ampicillin should be given intravenously. This should be continued for 7 days and in the meantime the patient observed to see whether haemodialysis might be necessary.

The prevention of leptospirosis is difficult, as there is such a large animal reservoir. For military personnel in highly endemic areas, doxycycline 200 mg once a week has been shown to be a very effective prophylaxis.

In summary, even if initial antibody tests are negative leptospirosis should be suspected in an illness characterized by headache, abdominal pain, jaundice and thrombocytopenia and therapy should be given empirically after appropriate cultures have been taken.

Further reading

WATT, G., TUARZON, M. L., SANTIAGO, E. *et al* (1988) Placebo-controlled trial of intravenous penicillin for severe and late leptospirosis. *Lancet*, **1**, 433–435.

Case 52 A young man with a sore throat and pulmonary nodules

A 17-year-old man who was previously well was admitted to hospital with a 9-day history of sore throat, fever, rigors and non-productive cough. On examination he appeared septic with blood pressure 130/90 mmHg, pulse 125/min and temperature 39°C. The tonsils were enlarged and covered with a white-grey exudate and there was tenderness to palpation anterior to the right sternocleidomastoid muscle. There was a left systolic ejection murmur on cardiac auscultation. Chest X-ray showed bilateral nodular densities suggestive of pulmonary abscesses. Laboratory investigation showed: WBC 13×10^9/l with neutrophilia and left-shift, Hb 12 g/dl and platelets 200×10^9/l. Liver function tests showed mild elevation of bilirubin and liver enzymes. The patient had been started on flucloxacillin and gentamicin. Blood cultures drawn on admission were positive after 2 days incubation in the anaerobic bottles. Gram-stain showed slender, tapering gram-negative rods with occasional spherical swellings.

Questions

1. What diagnosis was being entertained prior to the blood culture result?
2. The organism was identified as *Fusobacterium necrophorum*. What is the diagnosis?
3. What is the possible complication causing tenderness along the anterior border of sternocleidomastoid?
4. What is the optimal antimicrobial therapy?
5. What is the prognosis?

Answers

1. Based on the information provided in the case, the choice of flucloxacillin plus gentamicin suggests that a diagnosis of right-sided endocarditis caused by *S. aureus* was being considered. The patient should be questioned and examined to elucidate evidence for possible intravenous drug abuse.
2. The clinical syndrome described, that of a previously well

young adult with fever and pulmonary symptoms after pharyngitis, suggests right-sided endocarditis or Lemierre's disease. The finding of *F. necrophorum* bacteraemia confirms the diagnosis as the latter. Lemierre's disease was first described as 'post-anginal sepsis' in 1936. It is a specific syndrome due to *F. necrophorum* bacteraemia after oropharyngeal infection with distant metastatic foci secondary to septic jugular vein thrombophlebitis. This disease is uncommon and early consideration and diagnosis are vital to minimize serious morbidity. *F. necrophorum* is an anaerobic Gram-negative rod and is a normal resident of the oropharynx, gastrointestinal and female genital tracts and all may serve as a portal of entry into the blood. This disease arises on a background of pharyngotonsillar sepsis which may not be very evident at the time of admission to hospital and hence a suggestive history of such preceding infection is vital.

3. Septic thrombophlebitis of the internal jugular vein has been well described in this syndrome and is suggested by lateral neck pain and tenderness along the anterior border of the steinocleidomastoid muscle. A mass may be palpable, but local findings may be absent. Other complications arising from septic emboli include pulmonary abscess, septic arthritis and splenic abscess, and death may ensue from fulminant sepsis.

4. The optimal antimicrobial regimen is uncertain, however occasional isolates are resistant to penicillin. Metronidazole or cefoxitin are quite useful and therapy should be continued for a minimum of 6 weeks. In the initial stages where the diagnosis has not been confirmed, metronidazole can be added to the empirical cover for right-sided endocarditis (the major differential diagnosis).

5. Early medical intervention with specific antimicrobial therapy usually results in full recovery. Ligation of the internal jugular vein may occasionally be required.

Further reading

MORENO, S., GARCÍA ALTOZANO, J., PINILLA, B. *et al.* (1989) Lemierre's disease: post-anginal bacteraemia and pulmonary involvement caused by *Fusobacterium necrophorum. Rev. Infec. Dis.*, **11**, 319–324.

Case 53 Skin rash and peripheral neuropathy

A 38-year-old company director went to see her general practitioner because she was worried that her hands were becoming intensely white during cold weather. It would take some time for her hands to regain their normal colour, and this was accompanied by severe pain. She incidentally mentioned some numbness at the bottom of the left foot and 2 weeks later she returned with a complaint that the bottom of the right foot had also become numb. On the day of her second GP visit, a purpuric rash erupted over both legs and she was sent immediately to the dermatology outpatient department. A skin biopsy confirmed a leucocytoclastic vasculitis and she was admitted to hospital for investigation. She had no history of previous illness, except for an operation for gallstones 7 years ago during which she received 2 units of blood. On examination she appeared well apart from the purpuric rash, with a pulse of 80/min, blood pressure 110/80 mmHg. She was apyrexial. Examination of the chest and abdomen was normal.

On neurological examination there was a diminution to pinprick and temperature sensation up to the left knee and also up to the right ankle. The ankle jerks were absent bilaterally. Great toe dorsiflexion was graded 4/5 (MRC scale) bilaterally. One week later a patch of numbness appeared over the front of the right thigh and 3 days later another patch of numbness developed over the lateral part of the left forearm.

Laboratory investigations showed Hb 14.0 g/dl, WBC 5.0×10^9/l, platelets 340×10^9/l, ESR 3 mm/h. Liver enzymes were normal apart from an elevated gamma GT at 71 IU/l. Rheumatoid factor was positive (1:640) and antinuclear factor was negative. Chest X-ray, CT of the abdomen and a white cell scan were all normal. A test for HIV antibodies was negative.

EMG confirmed an asymmetric sensory/motor polyneuropathy, and further studies 3 weeks later confirmed a pattern of scattered reinnervation.

Question

1. What is the probable diagnosis?

Answer

1. Essential mixed cryoglobulinaemia secondary to transfusion acquired hepatitis C.

Comment

The combination of cutaneous vasculitis, Raynaud's phenomenon and peripheral neuropathy with a positive rheumatoid factor is a characteristic picture of cryoglobulinaemia. This could be confirmed by measuring cryoglobulins, and the C3 component of complement would be found to be low. Cryoglobulins are usually circulating immune complexes consisting of an IgG and an IgM molecule, and the IgM usually possesses rheumatoid factor activity. These complexes precipitate in the cold, which is why vasculitis occurs in superficial areas. Other features of cryoglobulinaemia (not present in this case), can be fever, arthralgia, hepatosplenomegaly, renal failure and nephrotic syndrome.

Causes of cryglobulinaemia include chronic infections such as hepatitis B and these should be excluded. In this case, extensive investigations did not reveal an occult fungal or bacterial infection and blood products have been screened for hepatitis B for many years. This is a case of hepatitis C infection for which blood screening was not introduced until 1990 (after her transfusion). The only clue to liver disease in this case is the slightly elevated gamma GT but persistent hepatitis C infection may be accompanied by completely normal liver function tests.

The hepatitis C virus was discovered through molecular biology techniques and it has not yet been cultured. Therefore, molecular biology techniques remain important in managing the patient. The polymerase chain reaction (PCR) can be used to amplify minute amounts of circulating viral RNA and kits are available which can quantify the amount of virus in the circulation. This technique will be very useful in assessing response to treatment and allowing anti-viral therapy to be tailored to each patient's need in the future.

The treatment for hepatitis C infection is interferon alfa and around 80% of patients who receive it develop normal transaminases during the course of therapy. A sustained response is defined as the occurrence of normal liver function tests and no virus detectable in the blood by PCR more than 12 months after stopping treatment. A sustained response is seen in 25% of cases after interferon therapy and it seems that late relapses after this are very rare. In the future, it may be that those with virus of genotype lb will receive a higher dose of interferon than the currently used 3MU three times a week, but those with the more sensitive variants such as la and 3 may be given standard treatment.

Not only does the genotype of hepatitis C virus affect the response of therapy, but so does the duration of infection, and this may be because the virus adapts to the host by mutations. In the case of hepatitis B, it is known that mutations can change T cell epitopes leading to immune avoidance, and a similar situation might occur in hepatitis C infection.

A particular difficulty in the future will be simultaneous infection with hepatitis C and HIV. Hepatitis B is very common in patients with AIDS, but because the damage produced by hepatitis B is immune mediated, levels of transaminases fall as the immunosuppression progresses. However, the patients are more likely to become chronic carriers of hepatitis B and have less response to interferon. Because hepatitis C seems to damage the liver directly rather than through immune mechanisms, hepatitis C can be rapidly progressive in HIV. In fact, the liver disease may cause the death of a patient before the other complications of HIV disease set in. Interferon therapy will produce a good response in these patients but at the expense of depressing the CD4 count even further.

Another difficult group of patients to treat may be haemophiliacs, who probably have numerous serotypes of hepatitis C virus in the circulation because of repeated transfusions in the past. Interferon therapy may control some of the genotypes but not others.

One of controversial issues in hepatitis C research is whether or not a liver biopsy should be obtained before commencing treatment with interferon. It has been shown that liver fibrosis can be present even in the face of normal liver function tests, and of patients who are positive for hepatitis C antibodies, 90% will have some form of liver damage. Some centres offer an initial liver biopsy and perform a biopsy again at the end of 6 or 9 months of interferon treatment. If no liver fibrosis is found on the first biopsy then no interferon treatment is given. This issue is still highly controversial, given the risks inherent in liver biopsy.

As interferon produces a sustained response in only 25% of

patients, other agents have been considered as treatment for hepatitis C. In particular, ribavirin, a nucleoside analogue, has been used in some patients for 1 year without any side-effects and it is usually used in combination with interferon. This approach seems to give a long-term response rate of around 50% and may become standard practice in the future. However, results from trials can be very slow and research is hampered to a great extent by the lack of an animal model and an inability to grow the virus in the laboratory.

Interferon alfa is a naturally occurring substance, produced in response to viral infections and therefore it is not surprising that the side-effects of interferon are described as 'flu-like'. Bone marrow suppression may occur, and there have been cardiovascular problems such as low blood pressure, high blood pressure and arrhythmias. Hepatoxicity has also occurred. An interesting side-effect of interferon alfa is the exacerbation of thyroid autoimmunity. A recent study showed that 12% of hepatitis C patients were positive for thyroid autoantibodies. Various thyroid-related problems were seen following interferon treatment in those positive patients such as subclinical hypothyroidism, thyrotoxicosis and increased titres of thyroid antibodies. Interferon alfa did not induce thyroid autoimmunity in autoantibody-negative patients. It may be wise, therefore, to measure thyroid function and autoantibody status before the start of therapy.

Several patients infected with hepatitis C seem to have developed Sjögren's syndrome, and a recent prospective study of 10 patients with primary Sjögren's syndrome showed that four were infected with hepatitis C virus. This does not prove a direct link, but it does make a case for testing patients with Sjögren's syndrome for the hepatitis C virus. This is especially true in cases of Sjögren's syndrome associated with cryoglobulinaemia.

Further reading

AGNELLO, V., CHUNG, R. T. and KAPLAN, L. M. (1992) A role for hepatitis C virus in infection in type II cryoglobulinaemia. *N. Engl. J. Med.*, **327**, 1490–1495.

Index